Catheterization Hemodynamics

Guest Editor

MICHAEL J. LIM, MD

CARDIOLOGY CLINICS

www.cardiology.theclinics.com

Consulting Editor
MICHAEL H. CRAWFORD, MD

May 2011 • Volume 29 • Number 2

SAUNDERS an imprint of ELSEVIER, Inc.

W.B. SAUNDERS COMPANY
A Division of Elsevier Inc.

1600 John F. Kennedy Blvd. • Suite 1800 • Philadelphia, PA 19103-2899

http://www.theclinics.com

CARDIOLOGY CLINICS Volume 29, Number 2
May 2011 ISSN 0733-8651, ISBN-13: 978-1-4557-0425-5

Editor: Barbara Cohen-Kligerman
Developmental Editor: Donald E. Mumford

Cardiology Clinics (ISSN 0733-8651) is published quarterly by Elsevier Inc., 360 Park Avenue South, New York, NY 10010-1710. Months of issue are February, May, August, and November. Business and Editorial Offices: 1600 John F. Kennedy Blvd., Ste. 1800, Philadelphia, PA 19103-2899. Customer Service Office: 3251 Riverport Lane, Maryland Heights, MO 63043. Periodicals postage paid at New York, NY and additional mailing offices. Subscription prices are $282.00 per year for US individuals, $458.00 per year for US institutions, $139.00 per year for US students and residents, $345.00 per year for Canadian individuals, $569.00 per year for Canadian institutions, $400.00 per year for international individuals, $569.00 per year for international institutions and $196.00 per year for Canadian and international students/residents. To receive student/resident rate, orders must be accompanied by name of affiliated institution, data of term, and the *signature* of program/residency coordinator on institution letterhead. Orders will be billed at individual rate until proof of status is received. Foreign air speed delivery is included in all *Clinics* subscription prices. All prices are subject to change without notice. **POSTMASTER:** Send address changes to *Cardiology Clinics*, Elsevier Health Sciences Division, Subscription Customer Service, 3251 Riverport Lane, Maryland Heights, MO 63043. **Customer Service: 1-800-654-2452 (U.S. and Canada); 314-447-8871 (outside U.S. and Canada). Fax: 314-447-8029. E-mail: journalscustomerservice-usa@elsevier.com (for print support); journalsonlinesupport-usa@ elsevier.com (for online support).**

Reprints. For copies of 100 or more, of articles in this publication, please contact the Commercial Reprints Department, Elsevier Inc., 360 Park Avenue South, New York, NY 10010-1710. Tel.: 212-633-3812; Fax: 212-462-1935; E-mail: reprints@elsevier.com.

Cardiology Clinics is also published in Spanish by McGraw-Hill Interamericana Editores S. A., P.O. Box 5-237, 06500, Mexico D. F., Mexico; in Portuguese by Reichmann and Alfonso Editores Rio de Janeiro, Brazil; and in Greek by Dimitrios P. Lagos, 8 Pondon Street, GR115-28 Ilissia, Greece.

Cardiology Clinics is covered in *MEDLINE/PubMed (Index Medicus), Excerpta Medica, The Cumulative Index to Nursing and Allied Health Literature* (CINAHL).

Printed and bound by CPI Group (UK) Ltd, Croydon, CR0 4YY

Transferred to Digital Print 2011

Contributors

CONSULTING EDITOR

MICHAEL H. CRAWFORD, MD
Professor of Medicine, University of California,
San Francisco; Lucie Stern Chair in Cardiology
and Chief of Clinical Cardiology, University
of California, San Francisco Medical Center,
San Francisco, California

GUEST EDITOR

MICHAEL J. LIM, MD, FACC, FSCAI
Director, Division of Cardiology and J. Gerard
Mudd Cardiac Catheterization Laboratory;
Associate Professor of Medicine, Department
of Internal Medicine, Saint Louis University
School of Medicine, St Louis, Missouri

AUTHORS

AMR ABBAS, MD
Division of Cardiovascular Medicine, William
Beaumont Hospital, Royal Oak, Michigan

BARRY A. BORLAUG, MD
Associate Professor of Medicine, Division
of Cardiovascular Diseases, Department
of Medicine, Mayo Clinic and Foundation,
Rochester, Minnesota

ROBERT C. BOURGE, MD
Professor of Medicine, Radiology, and
Surgery; and Director, Division of
Cardiovascular Diseases, Department of
Medicine, University of Alabama at
Birmingham, Birmingham, Alabama

NIRAJ DOCTOR, MD
Cedars-Sinai Heart Institute, Cedars-Sinai
Medical Center, Los Angeles, California

KEVIN P. FITZGERALD, MD
Comprehensive Cardiology Consultants,
Crestview Hills, Kentucky

GREGORY FONTANA, MD
Cedars-Sinai Heart Institute, Cedars-Sinai
Medical Center, Los Angeles, California

JAMES A. GOLDSTEIN, MD
Division of Cardiovascular Medicine, William
Beaumont Hospital, Royal Oak, Michigan

ASMA HUSSAINI, MS, PA-C
Cedars-Sinai Heart Institute, Cedars-Sinai
Medical Center, Los Angeles, California

HASAN JILAIHAWI, MD
Cedars-Sinai Heart Institute, Cedars-Sinai
Medical Center, Los Angeles, California

RAMI KAHWASH, MD
Assistant Professor in Internal Medicine,
Division of Cardiovascular Medicine, Section
of Heart Failure and Transplant, Davis Heart/
Lung Research Institute, Columbus, Ohio

SAIBAL KAR, MD
Cedars-Sinai Heart Institute, Cedars-Sinai
Medical Center, Los Angeles, California

DAVID A. KASS, MD
Abraham and Virginia Weiss Professor
of Cardiology, Division of Cardiology,
Department of Medicine, Johns Hopkins
Medical Institutions, Baltimore, Maryland

MORTON J. KERN, MD, FSCAI, FAHA, FACC
Professor of Medicine and Associate Chief, Division of Cardiology, University of California, Irvine, Orange; Chief of Cardiology, Long Beach Veterans Administration Hospital, Long Beach, California

CARL V. LEIER, MD
The James W. Overstreet Professor of Internal Medicine, Division of Cardiovascular Medicine, Department of Internal Medicine, The Ohio State University, Davis Heart/Lung Research Institute; Professor, Department of Pharmacology, The Ohio State University Medical Center, Columbus, Ohio

ELDRIN F. LEWIS, MD, MPH
Assistant Professor of Medicine, Cardiovascular Division, Department of Medicine, Brigham and Women's Hospital, Boston, Massachusetts

MICHAEL J. LIM, MD, FACC, FSCAI
Director, Division of Cardiology and J. Gerard Mudd Cardiac Catheterization Laboratory; Associate Professor of Medicine, Department of Internal Medicine, Saint Louis University School of Medicine, St Louis, Missouri

C. RYAN LONGNECKER, MD
Division of Cardiology, Department of Internal Medicine, Saint Louis University School of Medicine, St Louis, Missouri

RAJ MAKKAR, MD
Cedars-Sinai Heart Institute, Cedars-Sinai Medical Center, Los Angeles, California

ROBERT J. MENTZ, MD
Medical Resident, Department of Internal Medicine, Brigham and Women's Hospital, Boston, Massachusetts

LESLIE MILLER, MD
Walters Chair of Cardiovascular Medicine and Director of Cardiology Programs, Washington Hospital Center and Georgetown University Hospital, Washington, DC

ISH SINGLA, MD
Instructor, Division of Cardiovascular Diseases, Department of Medicine, University of Alabama at Birmingham, Birmingham, Alabama

PAUL SORAJJA, MD
Associate Professor of Medicine, Mayo Clinic College of Medicine, Mayo Clinic, Rochester, Minnesota

JOSÉ A. TALLAJ, MD
Associate Professor, Division of Cardiovascular Diseases, Department of Medicine, University of Alabama at Birmingham; Birmingham Veterans Affairs Medical Center, Birmingham, Alabama

ALFREDO TRENTO, MD
Cedars-Sinai Heart Institute, Cedars-Sinai Medical Center, Los Angeles, California

Contents

Symptoms and physical signs reflect distinct pathophysiologic derangements of anatomic components and mechanics, a construct that serves as the foundation for clinical evaluation of the cardiovascular system. Evaluation of hemodynamic derangements should be based on interrogation of a cardiac anatomic-physiologic approach to circulatory pathophysiology. This article illustrates a pragmatic problem-solving approach to 3 cardinal hemodynamic symptoms and clinical syndromes: right heart failure, dyspnea, and low-output hypotension. This treatise focuses primarily on the complementary roles of noninvasive and invasive diagnostic studies in clinical hemodynamic assessment.

Cardiac catheterization historically has been the principal diagnostic modality for the evaluation of constrictive pericarditis, restrictive cardiomyopathy, and cardiac tamponade. In many instances, the hemodynamic consequences of these disorders can be accurately delineated with non-invasive methods. However, cardiac catheterization should be considered when there is a discrepancy between the clinical and non-invasive imaging data, and particularly may be required for the evaluation of patients with complex hemodynamic disorders. This report describes the methods and clinical utility of invasive hemodynamic catheterization for the evaluation of constriction, restriction, and cardiac tamponade.

Since the development and refinement of echocardiography, this technique has, for some time, been the mainstay for hemodynamic assessment of the mitral valve. This article discusses the key components of the invasive hemodynamic assessment of mitral valve disease and illustrates their utility through percutaneous transluminal mitral valvuloplasty for mitral stenosis and the novel transcatheter mitral valve repair using the MitraClip for mitral regurgitation. Changes in left atrial pressure and waveform, mean gradient, and cardiac output are critical assessment parameters for both safety and efficacy. Invasive hemodynamic assessment is an essential complement to echocardiography for the optimal guidance of these procedures.

> Over the past two decades, echocardiography has replaced cardiac catheterization for aortic valvular hemodynamic assessment. In recent years, however, there has been a rapid evolution of transcatheter aortic valve technology and, with its refinement, there has been the increasing recognition of the value of transcatheter hemodynamic assessment in complementing the information provided by contemporary echocardiography. With an emphasis on transcatheter hemodynamics, this article reviews the symbiotic application of these assessment modalities pertaining to contemporary transcatheter aortic valve implantation.

> The pulmonary valve consists of 3 leaflets and is similar in anatomy to the aortic valve. It is the least likely to be affected by acquired disease, and thus, most disorders affecting it are congenital. The most common hemodynamic abnormality of the pulmonary valve is the congenitally narrowed domed valve of pulmonic stenosis. Pulmonary stenosis is usually well tolerated in its mild and moderate forms. This article discusses the clinical evaluation, cardiac catheterization, and echocardiography of pulmonary stenosis and pulmonary regurgitation.

> The first prosthetic valve was implanted by Hufnagel in 1952 in a patient with aortic insufficiency. Since then, prosthetic valves have evolved into various mechanical and bioprosthetic shapes and sizes. Despite the excitement surrounding the current development of prosthetic heart valves, surgically implanted valves remain the mainstay of current practice, and this article discusses the hemodynamic issues associated with the more commonly placed valves.

> The adoption of invasive coronary physiologic lesion assessment before percutaneous coronary intervention has become routine in many catheterization laboratories. In the last decade, numerous studies have demonstrated favorable outcomes for revascularization decisions based on in-lab coronary physiology in many patients. The use of coronary physiology in the laboratory has been identified as a class IIa recommendation for patients in whom the clinical presentation and supporting data are too inconclusive to make an objective decision regarding treatment. This article reviews pertinent concepts and studies of the more complex applications of translesional pressure measurements for optimal patient outcomes.

> Routine cardiac catheterization provides data on left heart, right heart, systemic and pulmonary arterial pressures, vascular resistances, cardiac output, and ejection

fraction. These data are often then applied as markers of cardiac preload, afterload, and global function, although each of these parameters reflects more complex interactions between the heart and its internal and external loads. This article reviews more specific gold standard assessments of ventricular and arterial properties, and how these relate to the parameters reported and utilized in practice, and then discusses the re-emerging importance of invasive hemodynamics in the assessment and management of heart failure.

The pulmonary artery catheter will likely earn a place in the history of medicine as one of the most useful tools that shaped our understanding and management of various diseases. An intense assessment of its application in nonacute and non-shock decompensated heart failure has been provided by the ESCAPE trial, a landmark investigation that showed an overall neutral impact of pulmonary artery catheter–guided therapy over therapy guided by clinical evaluation and judgment alone. The current guidelines reserve the use of a pulmonary artery catheter for the management of refractory heart failure and select conditions. The pulmonary artery catheter remains a useful instrument in clinical situations when clinical and laboratory assessment alone is insufficient in establishing the diagnosis and pathophysiologic condition, and in guiding effective, safe therapy.

The evaluation and management of volume status in patients with heart failure is a challenge for most clinicians. In addition, such an evaluation is possible only during a personal clinician–patient interface. The ability to acquire hemodynamic data continuously with the help of implanted devices with remote monitoring capability can provide early warning of heart failure decompensation and thus may aid in preventing hospitalizations for heart failure. The data obtained also may improve the understanding of the disease process. It is important for the clinician treating patients who have heart failure to become acquainted with this type of technology and learn to interpret and use these data appropriately. This article reviews the implantable hemodynamics monitors currently available.

The interdependence of cardiac and renal dysfunction has emerged as a focus of intense interest in heart failure management due to the substantial associated morbidity and mortality. Captured in the clinical entity known as cardiorenal syndrome, recent definitions afford discussion of the acute and longitudinal evaluation and management of these patients. This article discusses potential pathophysiologic mechanisms of cardiorenal syndrome, epidemiology, inpatient and long-term care (including investigational therapies and mechanical fluid removal), and end-of-life and palliative care.

Erratum

An error was made in the February issue of *Cardiology Clinics*, Volume 29, Number 1, in the article titled "Emerging therapies for atherosclerosis prevention and management" by Kuang-Yuh Chyu, MD, PhD, and Prediman K. Shah, MD, on pages 123–135. Page 123 did not list the correct affiliation address, which is Oppenheimer Atherosclerosis Research Center, Division of Cardiology and Cedars Sinai Heart Institute, Cedars Sinai Medical Center, 8700 Beverly Boulevard, Los Angeles, CA 90048, USA.

In addition, the affiliations listed for the authors on pages iii and iv were incorrect. The correct affiliations are as follows:

KUANG-YUH CHYU, MD, PhD
Associate Clinical Professor of Medicine, Department of Medicine, University of California, Los Angeles; and Division of Cardiology and Oppenheimer Atherosclerosis Research Center, Cedars Sinai Heart Institute, Cedars Sinai Medical Center, Los Angeles, California

PREDIMAN K. SHAH, MD
Professor of Medicine, Department of Medicine, University of California, Los Angeles; and Director and Professor of Medicine, Division of Cardiology and Oppenheimer Atherosclerosis Research Center, Cedars Sinai Heart Institute, Cedars Sinai Medical Center, Los Angeles, California

Cardiology Clinics

VISIT OUR WEB SITE!
Access your subscription at:
www.theclinics.com

Foreword

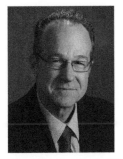

Michael H. Crawford, MD
Consulting Editor

As the cardiac catheterization laboratory has developed from a largely diagnostic role to a predominately therapeutic arena, operator skills in catheter-based hemodynamics have waned. This is an unfortunate state of affairs for several reasons. There are hemodynamic diagnostic areas where noninvasive techniques may not always provide a clear answer such as the distinction between myocardial and pericardial disease and the severity of valve stenosis. An accomplished cardiac interventionalist should know how to accurately evaluate these hemodynamic conditions. The significance of some coronary artery lesions can be unclear by angiography alone, necessitating a hemodynamic approach. Today the availability of percutaneous valve disease therapies necessitates a thorough knowledge of invasive hemodynamics to properly select patients and evaluate the success of the implantation. Finally, as more patients are developing heart failure due to a variety of causes, hemodynamic-based therapies are becoming more important.

For these reasons I was delighted that Dr Lim, a recognized expert in this area, agreed to guest edit this issue of *Cardiology Clinics*. He has selected an outstanding group of authors to cover this topic, including his mentor Dr Morton Kern. The new Cardiology subspecialty of Heart Failure has reinvigorated the hemodynamic management of cardiac decompensation. Thus, we selected a few articles previously published in the *Heart Failure Clinics* to complete the coverage of important hemodynamic studies in Cardiology today. General and interventional cardiologists will find considerable useful information in this issue of *Cardiology Clinics*.

Michael H. Crawford, MD
Division of Cardiology, Department of Medicine
University of California
San Francisco Medical Center
505 Parnassus Avenue, Box 0124
San Francisco, CA 94143-0124, USA

E-mail address:
crawfordm@medicine.ucsf.edu

Cardiol Clin 29 (2011) xi
doi:10.1016/j.ccl.2011.02.002
0733-8651/11/$ – see front matter

Preface

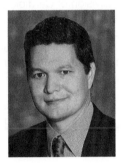

Michael J. Lim, MD, FSCAI
Guest Editor

This issue of *Cardiology Clinics* focuses on invasive cardiac hemodynamics. It is interesting to reflect back to the day when cardiac catheterization labs used to be the center of physiologic assessment for patients with valvular heart disease. The work done by seminal figures in the field regarding the accuracy of valve area calculation, the determination of cardiac output, and the ability to understand ventricular performance remains the backbone for much of what we take for granted in the modern catheterization suite.

The hemodynamics of cardiac and valvular performance have now become the domain of the noninvasive echocardiographic laboratory as Doppler waveforms can be utilized to translate blood flow velocities into the terms that we had familiarity with from the catheterization lab. More importantly, physicians could get the same data by noninvasive means; this was a major advance in clinical cardiac care. Simultaneously, the energies of the catheterization lab operators were focused on coronary artery disease, with Andreas Gruntzig's introduction of angioplasty providing a therapeutic option for patients.

The last year has seen a major advance in the completion of the first portion of the PARTNER trial, showing that an aortic valve could be successfully implanted in patients with severe aortic stenosis who were too high risk to undergo surgical valve replacement. This has once again brought a new and exciting therapeutic modality into the catheterization lab. Coupled with the early results and excitement surrounding percutaneous valve technology comes a renewed interest in the hemodynamics measured within the catheterization lab. In the present day lab, the operator must have a thorough understanding of the noninvasive and invasive hemodynamic parameters, as echocardiography and catheterization are complementary modalities in most of these patient care scenarios.

The articles in this issue aim to lend a present-day slant on the topics of cardiac hemodynamics. Drs Goldstein and Abbas start the discussion by exploring the critical importance of integrating the patient's clinical presentation, noninvasive evaluation, and invasive hemodynamic parameters for today's cardiac practitioner. This article then sets the stage for Dr Sorajja's discussions of the complex differentiation and discrimination between constrictive pericarditis, restrictive cardiomyopathy, and tamponade. It is exciting to have articles discussing mitral and aortic valve disease from colleagues at the Cedars-Sinai Medical Center that focus on the ability of catheter-based interventions to treat the underlying pathology and the hemodynamic findings associated with these cases. We have also dedicated an article to novel ways to understand and assess surgically placed mechanical valves as well as an article dedicated to the invasive assessment and treatment of the pulmonic valve. Finally, with the publication of the FAME trial, coronary

Cardiol Clin 29 (2011) xiii–xiv
doi:10.1016/j.ccl.2011.02.001

hemodynamics continue to gain momentum in current clinical practice. Dr Kern's article reflects upon the latest information for practitioners in understanding fractional flow reserve and its implications.

I must thank all of the contributors to this exciting issue and commend them on the careful and thoughtful work they did to produce a modern-day glimpse into the age-old tradition of invasive hemodynamics.

Michael J. Lim, MD, FSCAI
Division of Cardiology
Department of Internal Medicine
Saint Louis University School of Medicine
3635 Vista Avenue
13th Floor, Desloge Towers
St Louis, MO 63110-0250, USA

E-mail address:
limmj@slu.edu

Anatomic-Pathophysiologic Approach to Hemodynamics: Complementary Roles of Noninvasive and Invasive Diagnostic Modalities

James A. Goldstein, MD*, Amr Abbas, MD

KEYWORDS

- Hemodynamics • Invasive diagnostic modalities
- Noninvasive diagnostic modalities • Cardiovascular system

Symptoms and physical signs reflect distinct pathophysiologic derangements of anatomic components and mechanics, a construct that serves as the foundation for clinical evaluation of the cardiovascular system.[1–10] Evaluation of hemodynamic derangements should be based on interrogation of a cardiac anatomic-physiologic approach to circulatory pathophysiology. This article illustrates a pragmatic problem-solving approach to 3 cardinal hemodynamic symptoms and clinical syndromes: (1) right heart failure (RHF), (2) dyspnea, and (3) low-output hypotension. This treatise focuses primarily on the complementary roles of noninvasive and invasive diagnostic studies in clinical hemodynamic assessment. The anatomic-pathophysiologic foundations of this approach based on bedside physical examination have been previously published.[1–6]

CLINICAL ASSESSMENT BY ANATOMIC-PATHOPHYSIOLOGIC CORRELATES

The cardiovascular system can be simplistically viewed as a closed fluid system that obeys the rules of hydraulics and physics. Cardiovascular hemodynamic syndromes reflect derangements of cardiac anatomy and physiology and may manifest as either forward or backward syndromes. Forward syndromes may be grouped as hypoperfusion syndromes, manifesting early as fatigue and later as organ failure attributable to inadequate cardiac output (CO); similarly, syncope results from transient profound hypoperfusion. Backward syndromes attributable to right heart dysfunction manifest as systemic venous congestion syndromes, including peripheral edema, gastrointestinal-hepatic congestion, and ascites, whereas left heart dysfunction results in pulmonary venous congestion manifest as shortness of breath (dyspnea on exertion, orthopnea, and paroxysmal nocturnal dyspnea).

These symptom groups in isolation are nonspecific. Identical complaints reflecting disparate pathophysiologic processes can occur because of a variety of mechanisms. For example, dyspnea is an expected symptomatic manifestation of pulmonary venous hypertension attributable to a spectrum of left heart derangements, the

Division of Cardiovascular Medicine, William Beaumont Hospital, Royal Oak, MI, USA
* Corresponding author.
E-mail address: jgoldstein@beaumont.edu

Cardiol Clin 29 (2011) 173–190
doi:10.1016/j.ccl.2011.01.004
0733-8651/11/$ – see front matter © 2011 Elsevier Inc. All rights reserved.

underlying mechanisms of which vary greatly (eg, mitral stenosis, mitral regurgitation [MR], left ventricular [LV] cardiomyopathy). The treatments and prognoses also vary greatly. Dyspnea is also commonly of pulmonary origin, with circumstances in which the heart may be completely normal or affected only as an innocent bystander (eg, cor pulmonale). Similarly, peripheral edema and ascites reflect systemic venous congestion resulting from a spectrum of RHF mechanisms (eg, tricuspid valve [TV] disease, right ventricular [RV] cardiomyopathies, pericardial disorders). However, edema may also develop under conditions with normal systemic venous pressures, as may occur in patients with cirrhotic liver disease, inferior vena caval compression, and so forth. Thus, for cardiovascular assessment symptoms and signs must be characterized according to the underlying anatomic-pathophysiologic mechanisms, the next step to delineation of the specific cause.

CARDIAC ANATOMY, MECHANICAL FUNCTION, AND HEMODYNAMICS

To establish an anatomic-pathophysiologic differential diagnosis, it is essential to first consider the anatomic cardiac components (myocardium, valves, arteries, pericardium, and conduction tissue) that may be involved, and then focus on the fundamental mechanisms that affect each anatomic component, asking how such anatomic-pathophysiologic derangements and hemodynamic perturbations are reflected in the symptoms, physical signs, and invasive waveforms.

The purpose of the cardiovascular system is to generate CO to perfuse the body. However, although perfusion is the bottom line of the heart, the circulation is also a pressure-based system, with organ perfusion determined by arterial driving pressure modulated by vascular bed resistance. The regulation of the circulation (pressure and flow) can be understood by the application of Ohm's law. In classical physics applied to an electrical circuit, Ohm's law states:

$$\Delta V = I \times R$$

where ΔV is the driving voltage potential difference across the circuit, I is the current flow, and R is the circuit resistance. Circuit output or current flow thus is a function of the driving voltage divided by circuit resistance or $I = \Delta V/R$.

Ohm's law principles applied to the circulation are the foundation of hemodynamics, whereby:

Δ pressure = CO × systemic vascular resistance (SVR)

This approach can be applied to individual organ beds, such as the lung:

Δ pulmonary blood pressure = CO × pulmonary vascular resistance (PVR).

Alternatively, from a perfusion perspective, the equation is transformed, whereby:

CO = Δpressure/vascular resistance

The key components of blood pressure can be further considered. Thus,

CO = heart rate (HR) × stroke volume (SV).

SV is a function of 3 cardiac mechanisms: preload, afterload, and contractility. SVR is determined by total blood volume and vascular tone (a function of intrinsic vessel contraction or relaxation interacting with systemic and local neurohormonal influences, metabolic factors, and other vasomotor mediators, and so forth).

PERTINENT ASPECTS OF CARDIAC MECHANICS

The hemodynamic evaluation of the circulation may be considered as 2 sides of a single coin of cardiac function: systolic function, the ability of the heart to pump and perfuse; and diastolic performance, the ability of the chambers to fill at physiologic pressures with the preload necessary to generate SV.

Systolic Performance

Systolic function reflects the ability of the ventricle to contract and generate stroke work, a function determined by its loading conditions (both preload and afterload) and the contractile state. Systolic dysfunction then develops because of primary derangements of volume overload, pressure overload, or cardiomyopathic processes. It is important to distinguish depression of systolic performance caused by pressure/volume overload from primary contractile failure related to cardiomyopathy with damage to the contractile apparatus (eg, ischemic or nonischemic cardiomyopathies). Systolic dysfunction reduces SV, leading to low CO, resulting in fatigue and in most severe stages, organ hypoperfusion and hypotension.

Diastolic Function and Cardiac Compliance

Diastolic function is the ability of a chamber to obtain its necessary preload at physiologic filling pressures. Functional preload is the amount of blood distending the cardiac chamber. This volume is reflected in filling pressure according to individual chamber compliance. Compliance is a reflection of the relationship between diastolic pressure (DP) and volume in each individual cardiac chamber. There are 4 phases of diastole: isovolumic relaxation (IVRT), early filling, diastasis, and atrial contraction. In addition, because of the absence of valves between the pulmonary veins and the left atrium, diastolic motion during diastole has been shown to be limited during increased left atrial (LA) pressures and diastolic dysfunction. Under normal conditions, there is a defined IVRT, followed by mitral valve (MV) opening; most of the LV filling occurs in this early filling phase, through ventricular suction (lisotropic function); this is followed by equilibration of LA and ventricular pressures and temporary cessation of flow. Finally, there is atrial contraction, the booster pump function that atrial kick delivers additional ventricular preload; atrial booster pump function also optimizes ventricular filling at a lower mean atrial pressure, for the end-diastolic kick increases ventricular end DP as the atria actively relax (X descent), thereby facilitating ventricular-atrial pressure reversal, which closes the atrioventricular (AV) valves (atriogenic valve closure), minimizing the effects of ventricular DP on the back tributaries of filling (ie, the lungs).

Measurement of intracardiac filling pressures (eg, pressure at end diastole) is used for 2 basic purposes: to determine (1) whether there is increased pressure exerting adverse congestive effects and (2) whether preload is adequate to assist with appropriate forward ejection. With respect to assessing true preload, pressure is a convenient surrogate of chamber volume, which is exquisitely influenced by the compliance of the chamber being interrogated. Therefore, filling pressure reasonably reflects chamber volume and preload only if chamber compliance is normal. However, impaired compliance, attributable either to extrinsic influences such as pericardial disease or ventricular interaction, or intrinsic diastolic dysfunction associated with hypertrophy, infiltration or ischemia, or primary pressure and volume overload, influences compliance. In such cases pressure less accurately reflects true chamber volume. For example, LV preload may be markedly reduced but intracardiac pressures strikingly increased under conditions of cardiac tamponade or severe pulmonary hypertension (PHTN). Conversely, chronic volume overload lesion such as aortic regurgitation (AR) may result in dramatically increased chamber volumes, but when cardiac compensation is present, intracardiac pressures are relatively normal as chamber and pericardium dilate and become more compliant.

PERTINENT ASPECTS OF NORMAL PRESSURE WAVEFORMS
Relationship of Cardiac Mechanics to Atrial Waveforms, Venous Flow Patterns, and Respiratory Physiology

An appreciation of atrial waveform hemodynamics, the physiology of the venous circulations, and the dynamic effects of intrathoracic pressure (ITP) and respiratory motion on cardiovascular physiology is critical. Analysis of the atrial waveforms yields insight into cardiac chamber and pericardial compliance. The atrial waveforms are constituted by 2 positive waves (A and V peaks) and 2 collapsing waves (X and Y descents) (see section on normal pressure waveforms). The atrial A wave is generated by atrial systole after the P wave on electrocardiography (ECG). Atrial mechanics behave similarly to ventricular muscle. The strength of atrial contraction is reflected in the rapidity of the A wave upstroke and peak amplitude. The X descent follows the A wave and is generated by 2 events: the initial decline in pressure reflecting active atrial relaxation, with a latter descent component reflecting pericardial emptying during ventricular systole (also called systolic intrapericardial depressurization, a condition that is exaggerated when pericardial space is compromised). The X descent second component is affected by the pericardial space and changes when the ventricles are maximally emptied and therefore pericardial volume and intrapericardial pressure (IPP) are at their nadir.

During ventricular systole, venous return results in atrial filling and pressure, which peaks with the V wave, the height of which reflects the atrial pressure-volume compliance characteristics. The subsequent diastolic Y descent represents atrial emptying and depressurization. The steepness of the Y descent is influenced by the volume and pressure in the atrium just before AV valve opening (height of the V wave) and resistance to atrial emptying (AV valve resistance and ventricular-pericardial compliance).

Venous return to both atria is inversely proportional to the instantaneous atrial pressure, which is itself dependent on atrial compliance. The lowest return occurs when each pressure is highest. Normal IPP is subatmospheric, nearly equal to intrapleural pressure, and decreases during inspiration. IPP also tracks right atrial (RA) pressure and shows fluctuations that are associated with cardiac cycle. In general, the IPP increases when cardiac volume is increased and vice versa. Under physiologic conditions, venous return to both atria is biphasic, with a systolic peak determined by atrial relaxation (corresponding to the X descent of the atrial and jugular venous pressure [JVP] waveforms) and a diastolic peak determined by TV resistance and RV compliance (corresponding to the Y descent of the atrial and JVP waveforms).

IPP both approximates and varies with pleural pressure. The inspiratory decrement in pleural pressure normally reduces pericardial, RA, RV, wedge, and systemic arterial pressures slightly. However, IPP decreases more than RA pressure (RAP), thereby augmenting right heart filling and output. Under physiologic conditions, respiratory oscillations exert profound and complex effects on cardiac filling and dynamics. However, the effects on the right and the left heart are disparate, because of differences in the anatomic relationships of the respective venous return systems to the intrapleural space. The left heart and its tributary pulmonary veins are entirely intrathoracic. In contrast, although both right heart chambers are intrathoracic, the tributary systemic venous system is extrapleural. Normally, inspiration-induced decrements in ITP are transmitted through the pericardium to the cardiac chambers. On the right heart, these decrements in ITP enhance the filling gradient from the extrathoracic systemic veins to the right atrium, thereby enhancing the caval-RA gradient and augmenting venous return flow by 50% to 60%, which increases right heart filling and output. Because pleural pressure changes are evenly distributed to the left heart and pulmonary veins, the pressure gradient from the pulmonary veins to the left ventricle shows minimal change with respiration. Early diastolic transmitral filling pressure as well as LV filling are essentially unchanged throughout the respiratory cycle. However, left heart filling, SV, and aortic systolic pressure normally decrease with inspiration (up to 10–12 mm Hg), a phenomenon termed (normal) pulsus paradoxus or paradoxic pulse. By echo Doppler, normally during inspiration there is increased flow across the TV, with expiratory reversal of flow into the inferior vena cava (IVC) and hepatic veins.

Relationship of Cardiac Mechanics to Ventricular Waveforms

Invasive ventricular pressure waveforms reflect the effects of chamber preload, contractility, and afterload. The upstroke in RV or LV pressure (+dP/dT) is influenced by preload and contractility, but is a poor measure of either. Peak ventricular pressure reflects the ventricular afterload. Ventricular relaxation (−dP/dT) is an active energy-requiring process and reflects intrinsic aspects of myocardial contractility as the ventricle actively relaxes. Filling pressures in the ventricles

reflect diastolic properties, influenced by myriad factors both intrinsic to the chamber (eg, pressure overload hypertrophy, volume overload, ischemia, infiltration, inflammation), as well as extrinsic effects from the pericardium or contralateral ventricle through diastolic interactions.

ECHO DOPPLER APPROACH TO HEMODYNAMIC ASSESSMENT
Noninvasive Application of Ohm's Law

The noninvasive approach to hemodynamic evaluation using echocardiography with Doppler is based on the same Ohm's law principles, but derived from different parameters, because pressure, flow, and resistance are not directly measured. Instead, echocardiography Doppler interrogates velocity of flow, which is used as a reflection of either pressure or flow. Thus, the hemodynamic relationships are derived as follows:

Flow = area × velocity

Volume = area × time velocity integral (TVI)

$\Delta P = 4 \times (\text{velocity})^2$

Because in the absence of a shunt or significant regurgitation, flow across cardiac valves is constant, it therefore follows that flow across the aortic valve is the same as that across the LV outflow tract (LVOT). This concept is the basis of the continuity equation, the foundation of noninvasive flow assessment, whereby:

Flow1 = A1 × V1 = Flow2 = A2 × V2

Thus, echo Doppler, which directly measures area, velocity, and TVI, thereby provides correlates of pressure, flow, and resistance. For example, in aortic stenosis, an increase in resistance across the aortic valve results in an increase in ΔP between the LV and aorta by invasive measurement; conversely, by noninvasive continuous-wave Doppler, the decreased valve area is reflected by increased flow velocity across the valve.

The echo Doppler correlates of right heart hemodynamics are based on delineation of right heart anatomy and measurement of flow patterns, thereby establishing the anatomic-pathophysiologic correlates underlying clinical RHF. Echo delineates RA size, as well as RV size and contractile function. Echo Doppler hemodynamic correlates include the following:

A. RAP assessment, based on:
   IVC diameter and collapse with respiration: a dilated IVC as well as failure to collapse greater than 50% with inspiration (the sniff test) correlates with increased RAP.

Regional IVRT: an inverse relationship exists between regional IVRT as measured by tissue Doppler of the tricuspid annulus and RAP.

Ratio of the forward and reversed hepatic venous flow velocities: with increased RAP, there is more diastolic and less systolic forward hepatic venous flow with increased retrograde diastolic flow.

B. RV systolic pressure (RVSP) analysis: as mentioned earlier, the pressure gradient between 2 chambers is derived from the peak velocity across these chambers. This measurement is obtained by applying the Bernoulli equation. For estimating the RVSP, the peak tricuspid regurgitation (TR) is used. In the presence of a ventricular septal defect (VSD), the peak velocity across the VSD is used. By adding the RAP, the RVSP may be estimated.

RVSP can be estimated by 2 methods:

Peak tricuspid regurgitation velocity (TRV) through (4 × V2) + estimated RAP
Systolic blood pressure − 4 × (velocity across a VSD)2 + RAP

C. Pulmonary artery (PA) assessment: in the absence of pulmonic stenosis, RVSP is equal to PA systolic pressure (PASP). In addition, by applying the Bernoulli equation to the pulmonary regurgitation velocity (PRV), both peak (PRPRV) and end-diastolic (PREDV), we can derive estimates of the PA mean and DPs, respectively.

$$PASP = 4 \times TRV2 + RAP$$
$$PADP = 4 \times PREDV + RAP$$
$$PAMP = 4 \times PRPRV + RAP$$

D. PVR: increased pulmonary pressure may result from either increased PVR or increased pulmonary blood flow. With increased PASPs, an increased peak velocity of the TR jet occurs, as mentioned earlier. In addition, with increased PVR, there is decreased blood flow across the pulmonic valve. This situation manifests as truncation of the Doppler wave emanating from the RV outflow tract (RVOT TVI) occurs. Because PVR is the ratio of pressure to flow, a noninvasive measure of PVR may be estimated by the equation described by Abbas and colleagues[7-10]:

$$PVR = TRV/RVOT\ TVI \times 10$$

Noninvasive Imaging of Cardiac Architecture and Mechanics

In addition to providing hemodynamic correlates, echocardiography (as well as other noninvasive techniques such as transesophageal echocardiography, cardiac computed tomography [CT], and magnetic resonance imaging [MRI]) directly delineate cardiac anatomy, mechanics, and pathologic conditions. These imaging tools thereby provide crucial insights regarding atrial and ventricular size, LV and RV contractile performance, and valvular architecture, as well as direct delineation of pathologic conditions afflicting the chambers, valves, and pericardium. These imaging data, combined with the hemodynamic insights derived both by noninvasive and invasive techniques, facilitate comprehensive anatomic-pathophysiologic assessment of clinical hemodyamic syndromes.

ANATOMIC-PATHOPHYSIOLOGIC APPROACH TO DIFFERENTIAL DIAGNOSIS

Clinical hemodynamic assessment should be based on interrogation of cardiac anatomy correlated to pathophysiology. The primary goal is establishment of the pathophysiologic differential diagnosis, based on a synthesis of symptoms, history, physical examination, and integrated noninvasive and invasive assessments. To analyze each patient hemodynamically, it is essential to first consider each cardiac structure, enumerate the disease processes that may affect each structure, and then compile a differential diagnostic list of pathophysiologic syndromes that may manifest in symptoms. From a simple anatomic perspective, the components of the heart from outside in include the pericardium, myocardium, valves, coronary arteries, conduction system, and great vessels. Each of these structures may undergo various pathophysiologic alterations that result in a spectrum of specific hemodynamic derangements and subsequent symptoms related to those abnormalities.

Myocardial Abnormalities

There are 3 primary determinants of myocardial performance: preload, contractility, and afterload (in aggregate the determinants of SV). It therefore follows that all abnormalities of cardiac performance must be related to: (1) primary volume overload, attributable to valve regurgitation, shunts, or high-output states; (2) primary pressure overload caused by outflow obstruction or increased vascular (outflow) resistance; or (3) primary derangements of contractility as a result of ischemic or nonischemic causes. A dilated and depressed ventricle must result from either intrinsic cardiomyopathy, or decompensation attributable to primary volume or pressure overload. A dilated ventricle with intact contractility may result from primary volume overload (valve leaks and shunts) or high-output states.

As discussed earlier, diastolic dysfunction may be categorized as a result of intrinsic or extrinsic abnormalities. Intrinsic diastolic dysfunction may result from primary chamber volume overload (dilation and hypertrophy), pressure overload (hypertrophy and later dilation), or cardiomyopathic processes (eg, ischemic, infiltrative, inflammatory, fibrotic). Extrinsic factors leading to diastolic dysfunction include those mediated by pericardial restraint, septal-mediated ventricular interactions, or intrapleural influences. Diastolic dysfunction can occur with either preserved or depressed systolic function.

Diastolic function is influenced by myriad factors including the intrinsic physical properties of the chamber (eg, thickness, ischemia, infiltration, fibrosis), as well as extrinsic factors, including septal-mediated ventricular interactions, pericardial pressure, intrapleural pressure. Diastolic dysfunction results in abnormal chamber compliance, the result of which is a stiff chamber that has a higher filling pressure for any given preload. Impaired compliance (ie, a stiff heart) leads to pulmonary and/or systemic venous congestion, depending on which side of the heart is involved. Severe diastolic dysfunction reduces filling and results in chamber preload deprivation, contributing to low CO.

It is important to differentiate primary and secondary diastolic dysfunction. Primary diastolic dysfunction is designated as abnormal compliance with intact contractility (eg, with LV hypertrophy with normal ejection fraction). Primary diastolic dysfunction may cause pulmonary venous hypertension, resulting in symptoms and signs of congestive heart failure, and in the most extreme states limits maximal LV preload and impairs SV and CO despite normal contractility. Secondary diastolic dysfunction is that associated with ventricular systolic dysfunction. Impaired diastolic properties resulting from poor pumping performance lead to chamber dilatation, complicated by the primary myocardial insult (pressure overload, volume overload, or cardiomyopathy).

Valvular Pathophysiology

Valvular heart disease can be simplified into 2 categories: obstructive (pressure overload) lesions or regurgitant (volume overload) lesions. Obstructive lesions exert dual adverse effects, imposing increased afterload on the upstream chamber, delivering flow through the narrowed orifice and limiting preload or blood flow into the downstream chamber; they also limit the outflow into the downstream chamber and therefore reduce the preload or perfusion volume depending on the position of the valve in the downstream conduit. The effect of excess afterload on the upstream chamber is hypertrophy and ultimately dilatation and pump failure, resulting in higher filling pressures and less forward flow. Obstructions limit preload and therefore maximal SV and CO (preload deprivation).

Regurgitant valvular lesions result in primary volume overload of the chambers affected by the leak. In the case of semilunar valve regurgitation, the ventricle bears the predominant load. However, atrioventricular valve insufficiency affects not only the atria suffering the direct brunt of the regurgitant leak, but the ventricle itself, which must receive both the normal forward venous return as well as the excess recirculated volume. Regurgitant lesions result in chamber volume overload, predisposing to diastolic dysfunction; prolonged severe overload leads to systolic dysfunction. Even when ventricular performance is intact, regurgitant leaks may limit forward CO by compromising maximum effective forward stroke work.

Pericardial Abnormalities

Increased IPP exerts deleterious effects on cardiac compliance and filling. This situation is most commonly attributed to (1) primary pericardial disease (constriction or tamponade); or (2) abrupt chamber dilatation, as may occur with acute RV infarction. Regardless of the cause, increased pericardial resistance impairs chamber compliance, resulting in increased filling pressures. Abnormal cardiac compliance also limits ventricular filling with reduced preload, resulting in limited CO.

HEMODYNAMIC EVALUATION OF CARDINAL CLINICAL SYNDROMES
Hemodynamic Assessment of RHF

RHF results in systemic venous congestion manifest initially as peripheral edema. More advanced stages of RHF lead to bowel congestion, hepatomegaly (and cirrhosis), and ascites. There are numerous cardiac conditions with disparate pathophysiologic mechanisms that manifest systemic venous congestion. Furthermore, edema and ascites often result from liver disease or peripheral venous derangements unrelated to the right heart. Accordingly, peripheral edema and ascites can be attributed to RHF only under conditions of increased systemic venous pressure (JVP), usually related to RA hypertension. **Fig. 1** summarizes the anatomic-pathophysiologic approach to hemodynamic evaluation of RHF. RHF may also

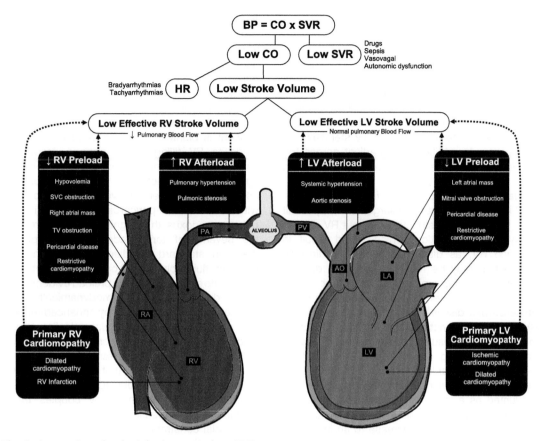

Fig. 1. Anatomic-pathophysiologic approach to RHF.

lead to reduced CO as a consequence of severe RV systolic dysfunction or increased RV afterload.

Increased JVP Without RV Enlargement

If the JVP is increased, the key to differential diagnosis is the presence of RV enlargement (indicated by physical examination by an RV heave [or lift] along the left sternal border, and easily delineated by echo documentation).

Superior vena cava obstruction

If the JVP is increased and the RV is not enlarged, then moving along the anatomic route from the distended neck veins toward the heart, the first possibility is superior vena cava (SVC) obstruction, characterized by increased mean pressure but an overall blunted waveform, particularly the Y descent which reflects poor flow from the great veins through the obstructed SVC, which also results in blunted respiratory oscillations. A pressure gradient between the cavae and right atrium confirms obstruction (eg, mass), in which case the preobstructive central venous pressure is increased, whereas pressure distal to the obstruction more closely reflects a normal RAP. Even

a small gradient across the obstructive mass can produce significant clinical problems. Noninvasive imaging studies, chest radiography (CXR), and especially CT and MRI, are typically sufficient and definitive, revealing the obstructive mass, and echo Doppler documents both the mass and impaired SVC venous return patterns.

RA hypertension

Excluding SVC obstruction, increased JVP directly reflects RA hypertension. Entities resulting in RAP increase without RV enlargement may result from RA space-occupying lesions (tumor masses, thrombi, and vegetations), in which the JVP pressure has a blunted waveform, especially the Y descent, reflecting poor transit of blood through the obstructive mass, and blunted inspiratory augmentation of right heart filling possibly with an associated Kussmaul sign. Noninvasive assessment with echocardiography should be sufficient and definitive in delineation of such atrial masses and their pathophysiologic effects.

TV obstruction

RAP increase without RV enlargement may be caused by TV obstruction (eg, rheumatic heart disease, carcinoid), which results in increased mean RAP with a prominent A wave/X descent reflecting augmented atrial contraction boosting flow through the obstructed orifice. The sharp X descent reflects accelerated atrial relaxation coincident with augmented atrial contraction. The blunted Y descent reflects poor inflow, resulting in impaired emptying of the RA. Imaging modalities can delineate the nature of TV stenosis and obstruction. In addition, the gradient across the TV, and hence the velocity, increases by Doppler.

Primary RV diastolic dysfunction

RAP increase without RV enlargement may result from RV diastolic dysfunction (without RV dilation or systolic dysfunction, which would result in enlarged RV, as discussed later). RV diastolic dysfunction may be related to intrinsic disease (hypertrophy, ischemia, restrictive, or other cardiomyopathies) or extrinsic effects as a result of pericardial disease. Regardless of the cause, RV diastolic dysfunction imposes increased afterload on the RA, resulting in augmented A wave/X descent, reflecting enhanced atrial contraction/relaxation attributable to increased outflow resistance into the noncompliant RV; the Y descent is blunted as a result of impaired RV filling. The RV pressure trace reveals increased filling pressure often with a steep increase to an increased end DP, which may inscribe a dip-and-plateau configuration (the square root sign), reflecting a stiff chamber. Restrictive cardiomyopathy (RCM) deserves special consideration, because the clinical syndrome is pathophysiologically and hemodynamically similar to and often indistinguishable from pericardial constriction. RCM, attributable to infiltrative diseases (eg, amyloid), radiation, and other inflammatory insults, results in increased RAP with a waveform characterized by an M shape with blunted components as a result of impaired atrial contraction and delayed RV inflow. DPs are increased and equalized throughout the cardiac chambers, there is RV dip and plateau, which indicates increased RV stiffness and mean RAP with inspiration (Kussmaul sign), a manifestation of inspiratory augmentation of venous return into the stiff right heart, which cannot appropriately accommodate enhanced preload. With impaired RV diastolic function, changes in the tricuspid inflow pattern suggestive of and similar to those of the MV occur (ie, impaired relaxation, pseudonormal, and restrictive). Impaired RV diastolic function is also reflected in increased RAP manifested as increased IVC diameter, decreased IVC collapse with inspiration, and increased diastolic reversal into the hepatic venous flow pattern.

Pericardial disease

RAP increase without RV enlargement may result from pericardial perturbations. In cardiac tamponade, the magnitude of JVP increase directly reflects increased RAP and IPP. The waveform is characterized by a prominent A wave and a sharp X descent reflecting enhanced atrial contraction into the RV made stiff by pericardial fluid. The Y descent is blunted, reflecting pandiastolic resistance to RV filling. In tamponade, inspiratory augmentation of venous return to the compressed right heart is intact. The resulting inspiratory competition between the ventricles for preload within the crowded pericardium is responsible for pulsus paradoxus, the magnitude of which reflects the severity of tamponade. Echo Doppler is the gold standard for diagnosis, documenting anatomic fluid including not only the size of effusion but also its effects on cardiac preload evident as RA and RV diastolic collapse. Hemodynamically significant effusions are indicated by enhanced respiratory variation in atrioventricular vale flows, with inspiration leading to an increase greater than 25% in TV flow but concomitant decrement in MV flow (the Doppler equivalent of pulsus paradoxus).

In constrictive pericarditis (CP), increased pericardial resistance more tightly couples the 2 ventricles and increases their interdependence. Pericardial constraint limits total cardiac volume; consequently an increase in filling on 1 side of the heart impedes contralateral filling through intensified septal-mediated interactions. However, in constriction, the heart is isolated from the lungs, resulting in lack of transmission of ITP changes to the encased cardiac chambers. Therefore, in contrast to cardiac tamponade, in which ITP is transmitted through the pericardium and inspiratory augmentation of venous return and right heart filling are intact, in CP, the inelastic fibrocalcific pericardial shell isolates the heart from the lungs, and therefore respiratory changes in ITPs are not fully transmitted to the cardiac chambers. Thus, constriction results in dissociation of respiratory effects on intrathoracic and intracardiac pressures, thereby inducing dynamic respiratory changes in diastolic ventricular filling and flow patterns and ventricular systolic pressures. However, the effects on right and left heart filling and pressures are disparate, because of differences in the anatomic-physiologic relationships of their respective venous return systems to ITP oscillations. On the right heart, the SVC and IVC are intrathoracic and the right atrium and ventricle completely intrapericardial. The constrictive pericardial shell neither fully facilitates inspiratory augmentation of right heart filling, nor accommodates whatever meager increments in filling occur.

Instead, the inspiratory gradient created between the extrathoracic systemic veins and intrathoracic but extrapericardial cavae, together with increased intraabdominal pressure associated with deep inspiration, augment venous return to the thoracic cage under conditions in which inspiratory augmentation of right heart filling is impeded by the constricted pericardium. The result is an inspiratory increase in JVP and right heart filling pressure (Kussmaul sign, the hemodynamic obverse of a paradoxic pulse). Anatomic-pathophysiologic relationships in the left heart are different. The pulmonary veins are entirely intrathoracic, the left atrium is not fully encased within the pericardium, because of the pericardial reflection around the pulmonary veins, and the left ventricle is fully within the constricted pericardium. Therefore, in constriction there is an inspiratory decrement in pulmonary venous pressure, which is not transmitted to the LV, resulting in reduced transmitral pressure gradient and flow velocity during inspiration. Because the cardiac volume is relatively fixed in CP, there is a reciprocal relation between left and right heart filling as a result of tight ventricular coupling. Therefore, the inspiratory decrease in LV filling allows a small relative increase in tricuspid inflow and RV filling. These disparate effects on ventricular filling lead to opposite directional changes in ventricular systolic pressures, with inspiration inducing an increase in RV but decrease in LV systolic pressure. This phenomenon, called ventricular discordance, indicates enhanced ventricular interaction and may be the most reliable hemodynamic indicator of constriction. As expected, the opposite changes occur during expiration, with increased left heart filling and reduced right heart filling, which decreases tricuspid inflow velocity and leads to diastolic hepatic venous flow reversals. In CP, the JVP is increased with augmented atrial contraction and relaxation reflected in prominent A wave and X descent. However, in CP, in contrast to tamponade, the first third of diastole is resistance free and thus the RA waveform manifests an augmented A wave and X descent, but a prominent Y descent, reflecting a pattern of late pericardial resistance. The initial third of diastole is resistance free followed by resistance to filling with a pressure plateau, inscribing an RV waveform dip and plateau, together with increased and equalized diastolic filling pressures.

Echo Doppler offers important insights into RCM versus constriction, based on assessment of LV thickness and architecture (eg, cardiac amyloid in which echo anatomic data reveal diffuse thickening and hyperrefractile myocardium), as well as flows, including mitral inflow velocity, mitral annular velocity, and hepatic venous flow. With restriction, there is increased velocity across the MV, reflecting increased LA pressure. Similarly, there is decreased mitral annular velocity. The E/E' ratio increases. Because the restrictive pathology affects the walls of both ventricles as well as the septum, variations in ventricular filling cannot be accommodated by septal shift. Thus, there is no ventricular interdependence. With inspiration, there is increased venous return, which in the setting of a stiff RV and increased RAP leads to inspiratory reversal of hepatic venous flow. Conversely, in constriction, the free walls are affected with the pericardial pathology, but not the septum. The variation in ventricular filling with respiratory variation is reflected by septal shift. With expiration and increased filling of the left heart, the septum is shifted to the right, with limited right heart filling and expiratory reversal of flow into the hepatic veins. The E wave is variable (higher with expiration and less with inspiration), but the E' is low.

Because RCM and CP are clinically and hemodynamically similar, imaging of pericardial thickness is critical to the distinction of constriction versus RCM. Because of a narrow field of view, even transesophageal echo is limited in evaluation of pericardial thickness. CT and MRI offer distinct advantages in imaging the pericardium. Although both modalities delineate pericardial thickness, MRI is superior, providing more comprehensive imaging with respect to its ability to characterize both pericardial thickness and the dynamic aspects of constriction and adhesion of the pericardial layers to the cardiac chambers.

Increased JVP with RV Enlargement

If RA-JVP pressure is increased and the RV is enlarged (obvious by physical examination as a palpable RV heave, or by ECG or MRI), the differential diagnosis now includes: (1) primary RV pressure overload, (2) primary volume overload, or (3) intrinsic cardiomyopathy (ischemic or nonischemic). The key to the differentiation of these abnormalities is based on the presence or absence of increased RV afterload, rarely in adults as a result of pulmonary stenosis and most commonly as a result of PHTN. Measurement of pulmonary arterial pressure (PAP) and PVR is easily documented by invasive study, but noninvasive Doppler measures of increased RAP, PAP, and PVR are also available.

RHF with enlarged RV but normal PAP

This syndrome results from either primary RV volume overload (caused by primary TR, pulmonary regurgitation (PR) or atrial septal defect

[ASD]), or primary RV cardiomyopathy (acute RV infarction or nonischemic causes). Primary volume overload lesions result in RA and RV dilation. Severe primary TR is characterized invasively by prominent RA V wave, with sharp Y descent reflecting rapid early emptying of the overloaded atrium; wide-open TR results in the RA waveform appearing similar to the RV pressure trace. Echo Doppler delineates TR as right heart dilatation with a prominent regurgitant jet by Doppler. There is increased systolic reversal in the hepatic veins with severe TR. Moreover, echo delineates that primary derangements of the valve may be discernible (eg, vegetation, rheumatic changes). In the setting of PR, color Doppler of the regurgitant jet as well decreases in the deceleration time of the PR Doppler waveform. ASD can be easily delineated by both two-dimensional and color Doppler.

RV cardiomyopathy resulting from nonischemic causes (which nearly always occur in association with similar LV abnormalities) is evident as increased RV filling pressures and noninvasively as RV dilation with depressed global RV performance. Echo reveals RV dilation and systolic dysfunction, and is often associated with secondary functional TR; there is typically concomitant LV dysfunction attributable to the underlying cardiomyopathic process.

Acute RV infarction results in severely depressed RV contractility indicated by a depressed, sluggish RV systolic waveform with diminished upstroke and amplitude, as well as delayed relaxation and increased RV DP. RAP is increased with RV dilation, but the acutely noncompliant pericardium results in a marked increase of right heart filling pressures. Abrupt RV dilatation within the noncompliant pericardium increases IPP, the resultant constraint further impairing RV and LV compliance and filling. These effects contribute to the pattern of equalized DPs and RV dip and plateau. RV diastolic dysfunction imposes increased preload and afterload on the RA, resulting in enhanced RA contractility that augments RV filling and performance. This finding is reflected in the RA waveform as a W pattern characterized by a rapid upstroke and increased peak A wave amplitude, sharp X descent reflecting enhanced atrial relaxation and blunted Y descent as a result of pandiastolic RV dysfunction. However, very proximal right coronary artery occlusions compromising atrial as well as RV branches result in ischemic depression of atrial function, which compromises RV performance and CO. RA ischemia manifests hemodynamically as more severely increased mean RAP and inscribes an M pattern in the RA waveform characterized by a depressed A wave and X descent, as well as

blunted Y descent. Acute RV infarction is hemodynamically similar to tamponade, but the diagnosis is suspected by its association with acute transmural ST elevation inferior myocardial infarction. The differentiation from tamponade is made obvious by ECG, which documents ST elevation MI and echocardiography, which documents the presence of severe RV dilation and systolic dysfunction, and the absence of pericardial fluid.

RHF from PHTN

RHF from PHTN is evident by increased JVP, an enlarged hypertrophic RV, evident on echo and associated with reversed septal curvature and a D-shaped septum bowing into the volume-deprived LV. RHF attributable to RV pressure overload often results in RV systolic pump failure with secondary RV volume overload. Under conditions of RV dilatation, the TV is vulnerable to functional incompetence, because the dilated RV tends to tether the tricuspid mural (septal) leaflet, rendering the valve prone to functional leakage. Secondary TR is common when the RV fails and enlarges as a consequence of PHTN, the increased afterload forcing the RV to preferentially regurgitate backward across the lower resistance TV, thereby perpetuating a vicious cycle of right heart dilation and low output.

Increased RV afterload leads to increased RVSP. RV outflow obstruction at the subvalvular and valvular levels is identified by a gradient between RV and PA systolic peak and mean pressures. Invasively, PHTN is indicated by equivalent increases of RV and PASPs.

Differential diagnosis of PHTN RHF caused by PHTN may be differentiated based on whether increased pulmonary resistance is precapillary, intrapulmonary, or postcapillary. Precapillary PHTN reflects primary abnormalities of the pulmonary arterial bed resulting from thromboembolic disease, primary PHTN, or occasionally extrinsic mass obstruction of the major pulmonary arteries from mediastinal tumors. Primary intrapulmonary processes include the broad range of primary obstructive or restrictive lung diseases. Postcapillary PHTN is attributable to increased pulmonary capillary wedge (PCW) pressure. Therefore, postcapillary PHTN resulting in right heart pressure failure can be determined through the same approach used for the evaluation of dyspnea, an algorithm based on why and how LA pressure is increased, as described earlier. Postcapillary PHTN caused by LA hypertension is suspected whenever PCW pressure is greater than 20 to 25 mm Hg. Echo Doppler is helpful in establishing the presence or absence of left heart anatomic (LA, MV, LV) derangements and dysfunction.

With increased PASPs, an increased peak velocity of the TR jet occurs, as mentioned earlier. In addition, with increased PVR, there is decreased blood flow across the pulmonic valve. This situation manifests as truncation of the Doppler wave emanating from the right ventricle (RVOT TVI). Because PVR is the ratio of pressure to flow, a noninvasive measure of PVR may be estimated.

Dyspnea can be ascribed to cardiac origin only if the PCW pressure is increased, typically greater than 15 to 20 mm Hg. If the PCW pressure is normal, then dyspnea must either be of primary pulmonary origin (eg, upper airway, lower airway, alveolar processes, parenchymal disease, pulmonary arterial problems) or related to a metabolic condition such as anemia. Accordingly, the differentiation of cardiac and noncardiac dyspnea is based on evidence of

anatomical-pathophysiologic perturbations that could result in increased PCW pressure (Fig. 2).

Using both noninvasive and invasive modalities, the diagnostic algorithm is based on interrogation of the anatomic course of the circulation from the pulmonary capillaries through the entire left heart. Accordingly, analogous to the anatomic-pathophysiologic approach to RHF, assessment of dyspnea proceeds along the course of blood flow (see Fig. 2): if PCW pressure is increased then cardiac dyspnea must reflect pulmonary venous hypertension. A simple anatomic approach reveals a limited number of anatomic mechanisms responsible for an increased back pressure, which may be found at the bedside and by invasive evaluation. Excepting the rare instances of pulmonary venoocclusive disease, pulmonary venous hypertension equates to LA hypertension, as a result of 1 of several mechanisms, including (1) space-occupying lesions (eg, myxoma) of the left atrium; (2) pressure overload

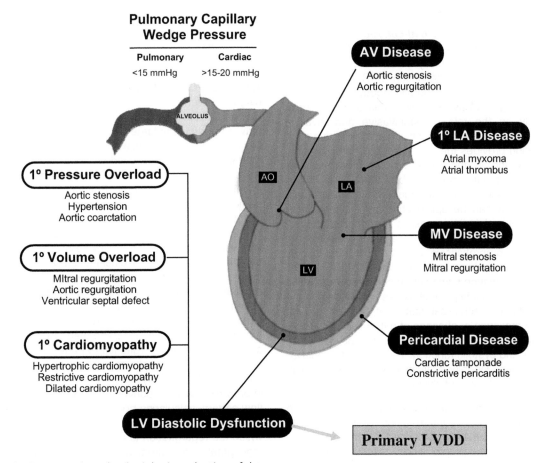

Fig. 2. Anatomic-pathophysiologic evaluation of dyspnea.

from MV obstruction or LV compliance abnormalities; (3) volume overload caused by MR or increased pulmonary blood flow from ventricular level shunts or high-output states; (4) intrinsic atrial cardiomyopathies, which may be ischemic or nonischemic.

Dyspnea with normal PCW If the PCW pressure is less than 15 mm Hg, then dyspnea is not attributable to a cardiac condition but more likely of primary pulmonary origin. However, several important caveats must be emphasized: (1) in some patients, chronic resting increases of PCW pressure greater than 25 mm Hg may be tolerated without resting dyspnea, as a result of thickening of the pulmonary capillaries, development of PHTN, and increased capillary lymphatic drainage of the lung; (2) PCW pressure may be normal at rest but increase dramatically during exercise or stress. Thus, in the dyspneic patient, if the resting PCW pressure is normal, hemodynamics should be measured during leg lifts, volume challenge, or after contrast administration; and (3) dyspnea may be also be an angina equivalent, a condition of myocardial ischemia that should be established by coronary arteriography.

Stepwise anatomic-pathophysiologic approach to dyspnea Evaluation of the patient with dyspnea requires careful synthesis of data from the history, physical examination, CXR, and serologic testing (eg, brain natriuretic peptide and arterial blood gas levels). However, this article focuses only on the role of noninvasive and invasive imaging cardiac diagnostic studies. Invasive evaluation provides the gold-standard hemodynamic data and in the modern noninvasive era has played a still important but often less critical role. Noninvasive interrogation of patients with dyspnea can be approached by the anatomic-pathophysiologic processes described. Echocardiography is the technique that provides the most comprehensive data and is most widely available, which may be further enhanced by other advanced imaging techniques (eg, MRI). These imaging techniques delineate the anatomic-mechanical status of the left atrium, the presence or absence of mitral valvular abnormalities that might explain dyspnea, as well as LV size and systolic function. Together with noninvasive echo Doppler evaluation, echo Doppler facilitates evaluation of dyspnea.

Assessment of the left atrium in patients with dyspnea Invasive interrogation of patients with dyspnea can be approached by the anatomic-pathophysiologic processes described in **Fig. 2**. The rare conditions of pulmonary venoocclusive disease or LA hypertension caused by space-occupying lesions are best established by noninvasive imaging studies (CT angiography and MRI). Generally, detection of an atrial mass (eg, myxoma) as the cause of dyspnea requires noninvasive imaging studies (echocardiography, CT, or MRI).

Evaluation of the MV In the absence of an atrial mass, the next anatomic site to interrogate is the MV, which if primarily to blame for dyspnea must either be obstructed or regurgitant. In mitral stenosis, invasively there is a pressure gradient across the valve that facilitates calculation of the MV area. The PCW pressure in a patient with mitral stenosis is characterized by a prominent A/X and blunted Y descent. Simultaneous LV-PCW pressure measurements show a pandiastolic gradient. In the modern era, this condition is easily diagnosed by echo Doppler, which delineates the anatomic calcification and fusion of the valve apparatus, diminished leaflet separation, and mitral orifice. Doppler assessment obtains the mean gradient by tracing the mitral inflow waveform, facilitating measurement of the pressure half-time derived from the deceleration time: The longer the deceleration time, the longer the pressure half-time, and the smaller the MV area.

In MR, invasive hemodynamics document increased PCW with a prominent V wave, the height of which reflects the degree of volume overload and LA compliance; if MR is acute, the V wave may be particularly large because the left atrium has not had the opportunity to stretch and accommodate to the volume overload. A prominent V wave may be reflected in the PAP trace, resulting in rabbit ears morphology. Patients with VSD, particularly acquired after infarction, manifest as increased PCW pressure with prominent V waves, the timing of the V wave peak may be delayed but the overall waveform pattern may be indistinguishable from severe MR. LV cineangiography distinguishes MR and VSD, as does oximetry across the right heart, which establishes the presence or absence of a left-to-right shunt. Noninvasive echo Doppler qualitative assessment of the amount regurgitation is performed by visual assessment of the regurgitant flow pattern. The regurgitant volume and the regurgitant orifice area are both calculated by using the PIZA phenomenon, which uses the convergence of the MR color flow pattern, calculating both the volume of regurgitation as well as the area of the valve through which the regurgitation is occurring, the effective regurgitant orifice area. Doppler also delineates the presence and locale of VSD.

Assessment of LV diastolic dysfunction If the MV is normal, then dyspnea caused by LA hypertension can be explained only by LV diastolic dysfunction imposing increased afterload on the left atrium. LV compliance abnormalities may reflect either intrinsic chamber processes (eg, primary LV pressure overload, volume overload, or cardiomyopathic processes) or extrinsic abnormalities related to abnormalities of the pericardium. Primary LV volume overload is induced by aortic insufficiency, MR, or ventricular level shunts (VSD and patent ductus artery). LV pressure overload may result from fixed outflow obstructions (aortic stenosis, coarctation), or dynamic obstructions (hypertrophic cardiomyopathy), or increased SVR caused by hypertension (± coarctation). LV diastolic dysfunction must also be viewed as occurring either with preserved LV ejection fraction or as a result of LV systolic dysfunction.

Regardless of the cause, LV noncompliance increases LV and LA DPs, because of inability of the ventricle to accommodate preload (venous return) without increasing filling pressures. LV DP may show not only increased mid and end DP with a prominent A wave (atrial kick), reflecting LV noncompliance of hypertrophy, fibrosis, infiltration, or external pericardial restraint. If LV and RV diastolic filling pressures are increased and equalized, differential considerations include increased IPP (tamponade, constriction, or as a result of acute RV infarction), RCM or massive acute pulmonary embolus. LV diastolic dysfunction results in prominent A wave/X descent, but there is no end-diastolic gradient on simultaneous LV-PCW tracings.

Under normal conditions, diastolic waveforms across the MV appear as follows: an IVRT, a rapid filling wave E wave, diastasis, and late filling A wave. Normally, more filling occurs early rather than late (ie, E wave is > A wave). By echo Doppler, early in diastolic dysfunction, there is an impaired relaxation of the ventricle, causing a delay in MV opening with an increased IVRT. In addition, less blood is delivered to the ventricle from the atrium in the early filling phase of diastole, with more blood available later in diastole (thus the A wave is > the E wave). With time, the increased blood volume in the atrium throughout diastole causes an increase in LA pressure. This increase leads to faster opening of the MV, which by echo Doppler is manifest as shorter IVRT, and an increase in ventricular filling volume and rate early in diastole through a high atrioventricular pressure gradient, with less blood left in the atrium at the end of diastole. This situation mimics the normal condition and is referred to as pseudonormalization. The E wave becomes greater than the A

wave again. In advanced stages of diastolic dysfunction, there is marked increased in LA pressure with earlier MV opening and markedly diminished IVRT, further increased LV filling volume and rate early in diastole with lesser contribution of atrial contraction, resulting in a restrictive pattern of diastolic dysfunction with marked increase in E wave velocity and decreased A wave velocity. By echo Doppler, LV diastolic dysfunction ultimately results in increased LA volume together with altered mitral inflow patterns. Early noncompliance is indicated by decreased mitral E velocity with increased A wave velocity (impaired relaxation). Subsequently, further increased LA pressure leads to increased E wave velocity greater than A level (pseudonormal). Progressive stiffness and increased LA pressure then results in increased E velocity but decreased A wave (restrictive). There is also progressive decline in mitral annular motion and velocity (E′). Increased LA pressure exaggerates reversal of flow into the pulmonary veins during atrial contraction with diastolic prominence of the pulmonary venous flow pattern and increased A wave reversal.

Assessment of LV systolic dysfunction Echocardiography provides excellent noninvasive delineation of LV systolic performance, including insights into both regional and global LV contractile performance. LV cineangiography provides similar information, but is less critical than before the noninvasive imaging era. Invasively, the LV systolic pressure waveform may reflect the severity of depression of contractility as indicated by diminished upstroke, reduced peak, and delayed relaxation. These derangements are similarly reflected in the aortic pressure waveform as diminished aortic upstroke, amplitude, and overall small SV. End-stage LV pump failure may result in pulsus alternans. LV systolic dysfunction results in dilatation and secondary diastolic dysfunction, resulting in increased diastolic filling pressures.

Assessment of LV afterload: outflow tract and aortic valve Dynamic outflow obstruction as a result of hypertrophic obstructive cardiomyopathy results in LV-aortic dynamic gradient, which may be present at rest and is shown by a pressure pullback from the LV apex through the body and LVOT into the aorta. An intraventricular gradient is located by carefully watching the slow catheter pullback under fluoroscopy, showing that the gradient occurs within the ventricle before it is pulled across the aortic valve. The arterial pressure waveform pattern often shows unique morphology, a spike and dome or bisfiriens waveform with intact upstroke, midsystolic delay, or notch, reflecting the obstruction and an overall small SV. In the modern era, echo Doppler is definitive, showing patterns of hypertrophy (eg, asymmetric septal), systolic anterior motion of the MV, and an outflow tract gradient, as well as associated MR.

Valvular aortic stenosis is evident invasively by fixed gradient across the aortic valve and a dramatic difference in aortic and LV waveform morphologies. The LV upstroke and amplitude are brisk, whereas in the carotid and aortic waveforms there is a depressed upstroke, and a delayed and diminished peak often with shudder findings, associated with low CO. The aortic waveforms are characteristic with aortic stenosis, revealing a slow rising and diminished amplitude, pulses parvus et tardus. Calculation of aortic valve area is well established by these techniques; the severity of the obstruction is reflected in the mean and peak gradients and CO. Echo Doppler facilitates precise analysis of aortic stenosis, delineating primary derangements of the valve (eg, bicuspid valve, or dense calcification with diminished leaflet excursion). Doppler allows calculation of the gradient across the aortic valve based on the Bernoulli equation. The mean gradient obtained with Doppler correlates well with that obtained invasively. However, the peak gradient is different. With Doppler, the maximum instantaneous gradient is what is measured. That is the gradient at the same instance between the LV and aorta, which is not necessarily the peak gradient of either cavity. However, invasively, the peak-to-peak gradient is measured. These measurements calculate the difference between the highest aortic and highest LV pressure. The aortic area is then calculated by applying the continuity equation.

In AR invasive hemodynamics reveal widened aortic pulse pressure and when decompensated leads to increased LV DP. In acute AR, the aorta-LV pressures are equalized at some point in diastole. The magnitude of AR is assessed invasively by aortography, revealing not only the severity of the leak but its effect manifest as LV dilation and later systolic dysfunction. By noninvasive echo Doppler, the LV is dilated and in later stages its contractile performance depressed. Primary derangements of the valve apparatus (eg, vegetations, prolapse, annular dilation, aortic dissection) may be apparent. The severity of AR is assessed visually as well as the PIZA and continuity equation. Assessment of the severity of AR can be performed by color Doppler by measuring the width of the regurgitation jet. In addition, the slope of the Doppler waveform (ie, the pressure half-time) is shortened in cases of advanced AR.

Evaluation of the Syndrome of Low-CO Hypotension

Investigation of hypotension is based on Ohm's law as applied to the circulation, whereby BP = CO × SVR. Accordingly, low-output hypotension must be explained either by diminished CO, low SVR, or both. Specific contributing mechanisms involve the determinants of CO and SVR. CO is a function of HR and SV, the last determined by ventricular preload, contractility, and afterload. SVR is determined by total blood volume and vascular tone (eg, autonomic influences, drugs, sepsis, neuropathies) (**Fig. 3**).

Low-output hypotension because of arrhythmias

The first step is assessment of the physiologic cardiac rhythm. Under conditions of low output because of depressed SV, reflex sinus tachycardia is the expected compensatory rhythm; lack thereof suggests chronotropic incompetence, which contributes to hemodynamic compromise. If the patient has a 1° arrhythmia and/or chronotropic incompetence, restoration of physiologic rhythm is the first therapeutic intervention (eg, cardioversion or bolus antiarrhythmic drugs).

Low-output hypotension because of low SVR

In patients with low-output hypotension and physiologic rhythm, the next step is to assess SVR. SVR, determined by total blood volume and vascular tone, is gauged clinically by peripheral perfusion. Low SVR is suggested by distal extremities that are warm and pink with brisk capillary refill. In such cases, hypotension likely reflects factors associated with vasodilatory stimulation such as sepsis, autonomic dysfunction, overdose of vasodilating drugs, or peripheral neuropathies (eg, diabetes) and other neurologic disorders. Invasive hemodynamics documents diminished SVR with high output and low aortic pressure.

Low-output hypotension because of diminished SV

In patients with low-output hypotension and a physiologic cardiac rhythm, low CO can be explained only by diminished SV. An inadequate SV can be explained only by inadequate preload, poor contractility, or excess afterload. Analysis of SV should be approached according to anatomic-pathophysiologic principles, with a stepwise focus on each cardiac chamber, as well as for the heart as a whole.

Invasively, it is essential to consider compliance properties pertinent to preload assessment. Cardiac preload is the amount of blood distending the cardiac chamber. In assessment of preload,

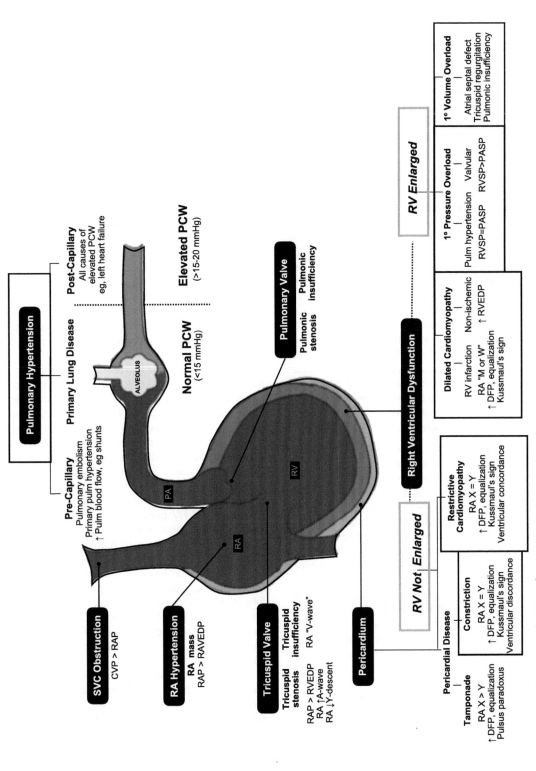

Fig. 3. Bedside hemodynamic evaluation of RHF.

measuring the chamber filling pressure is a convenient surrogate of chamber volume. The compliance characteristics of the chamber being interrogated have a striking effect on the pressure-volume relationship. Therefore, filling pressure reasonably reflects chamber volume and preload only if chamber compliance is normal. Because chamber compliance is influenced by numerous intrinsic (eg, hypertrophy, ischemia, infiltration, inflammation) and extrinsic (eg, pericardial pressure increases or intraventricular or intraarterial interactions) factors, it follows that there are numerous conditions in which filling pressure may be increased but preload limited. For example, LV preload may be markedly reduced but intracardiac pressures strikingly increased under conditions of cardiac tamponade or severe PHTN. Conversely, chronic volume overload lesion such as AR may result in dramatically increased chamber volumes, but intracardiac pressures relatively normal as chamber and pericardium dilate, become compliant, and compensate for the pathophysiology.

LV filling is the final common preload pathway that generates effective forward SV and thus CO. However, it is not uncommon for the LV to be preload deprived but other chambers to be overloaded. Thus, preload assessment must consider all cardiac chambers and conduits and be interrogated according to the course of venous blood returning to and ultimately delivered to the LV cardiopulmonary circulation.

Low output with decreased total blood volume Low output as a result of systemic hypovolemia is detected clinically by low JVP, orthostatic blood pressure changes, sinus tachycardia, and clear lungs. Invasive hemodynamics document diminished RA, PCW, and LV diastolic filling pressures. If LV function is intact, the carotid and aortic waveforms reveal intact upstrokes with a small pulse volume. Volume administration restores filling pressures, increases CO, normalizes blood pressure, and resolves the compensatory sinus tachycardia (lower HR). If volume challenge results in dramatic increases in filling pressures without the expected increase in CO and blood pressure, then preload was not the predominant, but certainly may have been a contributing, factor. Persistent hypotension in such patients suggests intense primary vasodilatation as a result of drugs or sepsis. Echo reveals preload deprived cardiac chambers with preserved RV and LV contractility.

Decreased cardiac preload despite increased total blood volume
Right heart inflow obstruction Increased JVP exceeding RAP with a demonstrable JVP-RA

gradient indicates inflow obstruction at the level of the SVC or IVC; central venous waveforms proximal to the obstruction are typically blunted. Noninvasive imaging confirms the site and nature of obstruction. Increased RAP exceeding RV DP with an end-diastolic RA-RV gradient indicates either a space-occupying RA mass lesion or TV obstruction. RA mass lesions manifest an overall blunted RA waveform. TV obstruction results in a prominent A wave with sharp X descent resulting from enhanced atrial contraction/relaxation against the stenotic valve, with blunted Y descent reflecting impaired RV inflow. Matched and increased RA and RV filling pressures may indicate primary RV diastolic dysfunction. The differential diagnosis includes primary RV derangements (pressure overload, volume overload, or cardiomyopathy) or pericardial disease. Increased equalized DPs throughout the cardiac chambers with RV dip-and-plateau configuration suggest either constriction, restriction, or acute RV infarction. The differentiation of these entities is discussed earlier in the section on RHF. Overall, echo Doppler is a superior technique for elucidating these problems, rendering invasive evaluation often unnecessary to establish the diagnosis.

Decreased RV outflow Increased right heart filling pressures with normal or low PCW pressure indicates impaired delivery of preload from right heart to left heart, attributable to (1) RV systolic dysfunction (eg, RV infarction), (2) excess RV afterload because of outflow obstruction (at the level of the outflow tract or pulmonary valve), or (3) pulmonary arterial hypertension. Diminished effective RV SV limits LV preload not only because of reduced transpulmonary blood flow but also because of the effects of RV pressure/volume overload. RV overload can induce septal-mediated diastolic ventricular interactions, which adversely influence LV compliance and filling. Severe RV infarction depresses RV stroke work, leading to depressed transpulmonary delivery of LV preload. Thus, RV infarction with decreased LV preload results in a syndrome of hypotension, low output with clear lungs, and increased right heart filling pressures. RV infarction and its evaluation is discussed earlier.

Excess RV afterload is delineated by increased RVSP: RV outflow obstructions are evident by increased JVP with RV heave and loud late-peaking ejection murmur along the left sternal border. Invasively, RVSP greater than PASP suggests either subvalvular RV outflow obstruction or pulmonary valve stenosis. Clinical evaluation delineates PHTN, characterized by an RV heave and loud P2. Invasive assessment documents increased RVSP = PASPs. The magnitude of PA DP increase is dependent on the mechanism of PHTN. Calculated pulmonary resistance is increased and reflects the magnitude of obstruction in the pulmonary bed. If attributable to left heart cause, PHTN is associated with increased PCW. These entities and their differentiation are discussed in the sections on RHF and dyspnea.

Left heart inflow obstruction Under conditions of left heart inflow obstruction, reduced LV preload results in low-output hypotension despite expanded total blood volume, increased right heart preload, and increased PCW pressure. Inflow obstruction may occur at the level of the pulmonary veins, LA, or MV. LV preload is reflected by LV DP, which must be interpreted within the context of LV compliance. Increased PCW pressure with an end-diastolic gradient across the MV suggests either a space-occupying lesion in the left atrium or mitral valvular obstruction. The lack of opening snap and diastolic flow rumble on examination excludes mitral stenosis, and should lead to suspicion of an atrial mass or pulmonary venoocclusive disease. Noninvasive imaging is confirmatory. Increased and equal PCW and LV filling pressure indicates LV diastolic dysfunction, which may be primary (with intact LV contractility) or secondary (associated with depressed LV systolic function). Primary LV diastolic dysfunction reflects intrinsic LV abnormalities (primary pressure overload/outflow obstruction, volume overload, or cardiomyopathic processes) or extrinsic constraint (pericardial disease or intense ventricular interactions from the RV). Occasionally, acute LV ischemia with global paralysis of LV function may result in abrupt diastolic dysfunction with flash pulmonary edema and low-output hypotension LV contractility may be intact or depressed depending on the duration of ischemia. Severe LV diastolic dysfunction may result from a hypertrophic noncompliant cavity (eg, severe hypertensive LV hypertrophy, aortic stenosis, or hypertrophic cardiomyopathy), with increased filling pressures but reduced LV preload and SV further limiting CO. These entities and their differentiation are also discussed in the section on dyspnea (see **Fig. 2**).

Low output because of diminished LV outflow
Depressed LV contractility Reduced LV SV may be attributable to (1) impaired systolic performance, (2) decompensated primary pressure overload (hypertension or outflow resistance), (3) volume overload (mitral insufficiency, AR or ventricular level shunts) or (4) primary cardiomyopathies (either ischemic or nonischemic). It is important to differentiate contractile failure resulting from ischemic or nonischemic myocardial depression from pump failure attributable to chronic excess afterload conditions such as severe aortic stenosis. Regardless of the cause, systolic dysfunction reduces SV and CO. Transient acute ischemic LV dysfunction is excluded by coronary angiography. If present, severe left main or multivessel equivalents are noted and occasionally result in episodic low-output hypotension, often with flash pulmonary edema; more commonly LV contractility is depressed because of ischemic cardiomyopathy. These entities and their differentiation are also discussed in the section on dyspnea.

Depressed CO because of increased LV afterload Increased LV afterload impairs SV and CO, either with intact LV contractility or LV systolic dysfunction. Increased LV afterload can be categorized mechanically and anatomically as (1) dynamic LVOT as a result of hypertrophic obstructive cardiomyopathy, or (2) fixed obstructions as a result of subvalvular (membranes) or valvular stenosis or (3) postvalve level resistance attributable to systemic hypertension or aortic coarctation. These entities and their differentiation are also discussed in the section on dyspnea.

REFERENCES

1. McCullough P, Goldstein JA. Heart pressures and catheterization. Diagnostic cardiac catheterization. Blackwell Scientific Publications; 1997.
2. Goldstein JA. An anatomic-pathophysiologic approach to hemodynamic assessment. In: Kern MJ, Lim MJ, Goldstein JA, editors. Hemodynamic rounds: interpretation of cardiac pathophysiology from pressure waveform analysis. Wiley-Liss; 2009. p. 429–36.
3. Goldstein JA. Hemodynamic evaluation of dyspnea. In: Kern MJ, Lim MJ, Goldstein JA, editors. Hemodynamic rounds: interpretation of cardiac pathophysiology from pressure waveform analysis. Wiley-Liss; 2009. p. 445–6.
4. Goldstein JA. Bedside evaluation of low output hypotension. In: Kern MJ, Lim MJ, Goldstein JA, editors. Hemodynamic rounds: interpretation of cardiac pathophysiology from pressure waveform analysis. Wiley-Liss; 2009. p. 449–54.
5. Goldstein JA. Hemodynamic evaluation of right heart failure. In: Kern MJ, Lim MJ, Goldstein JA, editors. Hemodynamic rounds: interpretation of cardiac pathophysiology from pressure waveform analysis. Wiley-Liss; 2009. p. 455–9.
6. Goldstein JA. Cardiac tamponade, constrictive pericarditis, and restrictive cardiomyopathy. Curr Probl Cardiol 2004;29:503–67.

7. Abbas AE, Fortuin Schiller NB, Appleton CP, et al. A simple method for noninvasive estimation of pulmonary vascular resistance. J Am Coll Cardiol 2003;41(6):1021–7.

8. Lee KS, Abbas AE, Khandheria BK, et al. Echocardiographic assessment of right heart hemodynamic parameters. J Am Soc Echocardiogr 2007;20(6):773–82.

9. Abbas AE, Fortuin FD, Schiller NB, et al. Echocardiographic determination of mean pulmonary artery pressure. Am J Cardiol 2003;92(11):1373–6.

10. Abbas A, Lester S, Moreno FC, et al. Noninvasive assessment of right atrial pressure using Doppler tissue imaging. J Am Soc Echocardiogr 2004; 17(11):1155–60.

Invasive Hemodynamics of Constrictive Pericarditis, Restrictive Cardiomyopathy, and Cardiac Tamponade

Paul Sorajja, MD

KEYWORDS

- Pericarditis • Cardiomyopathy • Cardiac Tamponade
- Hemodynamics

Cardiac catheterization historically has been the principal diagnostic modality for the evaluation of constrictive pericarditis, restrictive cardiomyopathy, and cardiac tamponade. With the introduction of newer imaging techniques, there has been a shift in the evaluation of patients with these disorders to an initial approach of comprehensive noninvasive imaging after history taking and physical examination. In many instances, the hemodynamic consequences of these disorders can be accurately delineated with these diagnostic methods. Therefore, the hemodynamic assessment of these disease entities frequently can be made without the need for cardiac catheterization.

However, an invasive hemodynamic study should be considered when there is a discrepancy between the clinical and noninvasive imaging data. Although noninvasive modalities can diagnose these entities, there are limitations in their accuracy. Moreover, absolute intracardiac pressures cannot be measured noninvasively, and invasive catheterization is performed when this information is necessary. Because patients with straightforward conditions can be assessed primarily with noninvasive methods, there also have been an increasing number of complex patients with these disorders evaluated in the catheterization laboratory. Thus, there has been greater recognition of the need to obtain accurate and clinically relevant data from invasive cardiac catheterization.

PATIENT APPROACH

The hemodynamic assessment of these clinical entities should be individualized. Proper planning of the procedure requires a comprehensive differential diagnosis of the patient's problems, complete knowledge of the known data, the clinically relevant information that is required from the hemodynamic study, as well as the potential data needed in the event a diagnosis of restrictive cardiomyopathy (eg, pulmonary arteriolar resistance, ventricular biopsy) or constrictive pericarditis (eg, preoperative coronary angiography) is made. Vascular access sites and approach to gathering data should be delineated fully before proceeding.

Although all patients should be fasting for the catheterization procedure, intravenous fluids should be administered to patients who have a long waiting period after their last oral intake to prevent measurements from being taken during a low output, low volume state. Patients can be

Mayo Clinic College of Medicine, Mayo Clinic, 200 First Street South West, Rochester, MN 55905, USA
E-mail address: sorajja.paul@mayo.edu

Cardiol Clin 29 (2011) 191–199
doi:10.1016/j.ccl.2011.01.003
0733-8651/11/$ – see front matter © 2011 Elsevier Inc. All rights reserved.

lightly sedated but should be awake to simulate the hemodynamic milieu of their outpatient state. No parenteral oxygen should be administered before the procedure to allow measurements of oxygen saturations at steady state for calculation of cardiac output. Temporary pacing should be used in patients with irregular heart rates (eg, atrial fibrillation) to maintain consistent ventricular intervals to improve diagnostic interpretation of the hemodynamic data in these patients. If possible, continuous recording of hemodynamic pressures should be performed to allow retrospective review of these pressures throughout the study.

The accurate measurement of cardiac pressures with fluid-filled catheters requires the use of rigid large-bore catheters, with minimization of the tubing length between the catheter and pressure transducer. Fluid-filled catheters can reliably measure absolute and mean cardiac pressures. However, for analysis of pressure waveforms in patients who may have restriction or constriction, high-fidelity micromanometer-tip catheters (Millar Instruments, Houston, TX, USA) facilitate instantaneous recordings should be used. These catheters help overcome underdamping, which can mimic early rapid ventricular filling (**Fig. 1**). High-fidelity micromanometer-tip catheters are calibrated to fluid-filled pressures at baseline, and calibration is repeated after any catheter repositioning. Both 6 Fr or more multipurpose coronary guide and balloon wedge catheter (Arrow International, Teleflex Medical, Limerick, PA, USA) are relatively rigid catheters with large bores that accommodate 2 Fr high-fidelity micromanometer-tip catheters.

PATHOPHYSIOLOGY

Constrictive pericarditis and restrictive cardiomyopathy are distinct disease entities that can share clinical features and hemodynamic findings. However, because the causes and treatments of these entities are highly different, physicians must be able to differentiate the 2 conditions.[1,2]

Constrictive pericarditis results from pericardial inflammation, fibrosis, and possibly calcification that leads to loss of elasticity of the pericardial sac from scarring. Causes of constrictive pericarditis include radiation therapy, cardiac surgery, trauma, and systemic diseases that affect the pericardium (eg, connective tissue disease, tuberculosis, malignancy). The loss of elasticity impairs ventricular filling in mid diastole and late diastole, thereby limiting increases in ventricular volume after the end of the early filling period. The end-diastolic pressures become equalized or nearly equalized in all 4 cardiac chambers. The rigid non-compliant pericardium prevents the complete transmission of intrathoracic pressure to the intracardiac chambers. In addition, the total cardiac volume is fixed by the noncompliant pericardium. Because the ventricular septum is not involved, the ventricular septum bulges toward the left during inspiration and returns toward the right during expiration, leading to marked enhancement of ventricular interdependence. This ventricular interaction leads to reciprocal changes in filling and emptying of the right ventricle (RV) and left ventricle (LV).

Restrictive cardiomyopathy, on the other hand, is characterized by a nondilated rigid ventricle. The cause is frequently idiopathic, although desmin and troponin I mutations have been described in these patients.[3–5] Infiltrative cardiomyopathies, such as amyloidosis, hemochromatosis, and sarcoidosis, also can present with hemodynamics similar to restrictive cardiomyopathy. Radiation exposure also may lead to restrictive cardiomyopathy. Patients with restrictive cardiomyopathy or forms of similar cardiomyopathy have severe diastolic dysfunction with high-filling pressures in all 4 cardiac chambers and restrictive ventricular filling. Pulmonary hypertension also is common in these patients.

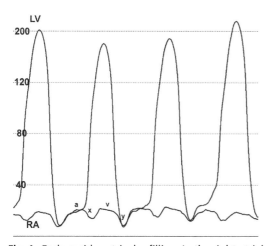

Fig. 1. Early rapid ventricular filling. In the right atrial (RA) tracing, there are rapid *x* and *y* descents. The *y* descent of the RA pressure tracing corresponds to the early rapid filling phase of the ventricular pressure tracing, which demonstrates the typical dip and plateau pattern. These hemodynamic tracings were taken using high-fidelity micromanometer-tip catheters from a patient with constrictive pericarditis.

HEMODYNAMIC ASSESSMENT

Both restrictive cardiomyopathy and constrictive pericarditis present with elevation of diastolic pressures out of proportion to systolic dysfunction. These hemodynamic abnormalities can manifest as a "dip and plateau" pattern in the ventricular pressure curves during early diastole and rapid *x* and *y* descents on the atrial pressure curves (see **Fig. 1**). Historically, the following criteria have been used for differentiating restrictive cardiomyopathy from constrictive pericarditis in the cardiac catheterization laboratory[6]:

- LV end-diastolic pressure exceeds RV end-diastolic pressure by 5 mmHg or more.
- Pulmonary artery systolic pressure is greater than 50 mmHg.
- In RV, the end-diastolic pressure is less than 0.3 of systolic pressure.

However, these criteria have been found to have poor specificity and they cannot be used as a single diagnostic tool to differentiate restrictive cardiomyopathy from constrictive pericarditis in the individual patient.[7]

Accurate assessment of constrictive pericarditis versus restrictive cardiomyopathy entails the use of both traditional and dynamic respiratory criteria. Respiration affects ventricular filling in constrictive pericarditis in a manner that is distinct from restrictive cardiomyopathy.

- In patients with constrictive pericarditis, the decrease in inspiratory thoracic pressure affects the pulmonary wedge pressure, but ventricular pressure is relatively

shielded from respiratory pressure changes by the pericardial scar. By lowering pulmonary wedge and left atrial pressure, inspiration leads to a decrease in pressure gradient for ventricular filling. Conversely, during expiration, there is a relative increase in the pressure gradient for ventricular filling. These findings are described as dissociation of the intrathoracic and intracavitary pressures (**Fig. 2**).

- In patients with constrictive pericarditis, enhancement of ventricular interdependence leads to discordant changes in RV and LV pressures during respiration. This discordance is caused by reciprocal changes in ventricular filling mediated by the ventricular septum (not by increased systemic venous return). These alterations manifest as reciprocal changes in peak systolic pressure, stroke volume, and pulse pressure in both ventricles during respiration (**Fig. 3**).

In patients with restrictive cardiomyopathy, neither enhancement of ventricular interaction nor dissociation of intrathoracic and intracavitary pressures are present. In these patients, inspiration lowers the pulmonary wedge and LV diastolic pressures equally. Therefore, the pressure gradient for LV filling remains virtually unchanged during respiration. Because there is no significant

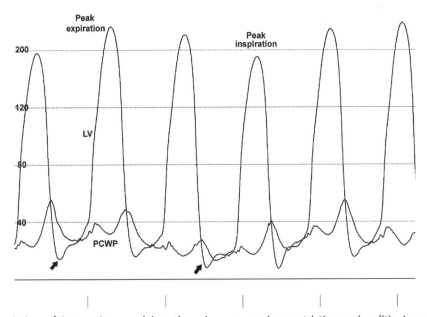

Fig. 2. Dissociation of intracavitary and intrathoracic pressures in constrictive pericarditis. In patients with constrictive pericarditis, inspiration leads to a decrease in ventricular filling by decreasing intrathoracic pressure relative to ventricular diastolic pressure. Conversely, during expiration, positive intrathoracic pressure leads to an increase in ventricular filling. These respiratory effects can be observed by examining the changes in the pressure gradient between the pulmonary capillary wedge pressure and ventricular early diastolic pressure (*arrows*).

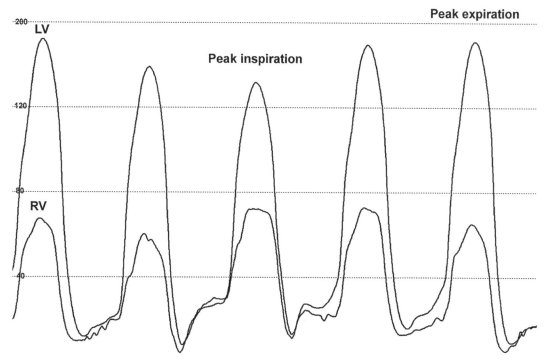

Fig. 3. Enhancement of ventricular interdependence. In patients with constrictive pericarditis, the total ventricular volume is fixed by the noncompliant pericardium. Thus, reciprocal respiratory changes in the filling of each ventricle occur. These changes are described as discordance in pulse pressure, systolic pressure, or stroke volume between the RV and LV during respiration.

enhancement of ventricular interdependence, the LV and RV pressures move concordantly throughout the respiratory cycle (**Fig. 4**).

Several studies have demonstrated the utility of dynamic respiratory criteria for differentiating constrictive pericarditis from restrictive cardiomyopathy. In a study of 36 patients, the presence of enhanced ventricular interdependence (ie, discordant peak LV and RV pressures with respiration) was highly sensitive and specific for constriction, whereas conventional static criteria were of no clinical benefit. To provide a quantitative means for evaluating ventricular interdependence, another study of 100 patients, which included 59 patients with surgically proven constriction, demonstrated the utility of the systolic area index (SAI). This method examines the ratio of the areas (mm Hg×s) under the RV and LV systolic pressures during inspiration versus expiration (**Figs. 5** and **6**).[8]

support the diagnosis of constrictive pericarditis at cardiac catheterization are the presence of epicardial fixation of the coronary arteries and pericardial calcification on fluoroscopy.

Equalization of pressures in all 4 cardiac chambers frequently is present in patients with constrictive pericarditis but is nonspecific because this finding may be present in restrictive cardiomyopathy. Moreover, disease states with volume overload leading to pericardial restraint can also demonstrate diastolic equalization and potentially significant ventricular interdependence. One recent study demonstrated findings of ventricular interdependence in patients with severe tricuspid regurgitation similar to that observed in constrictive pericarditis.[9] In this study, careful analysis during inspiration helped to differentiate the 2 disorders. During inspiration, patients with severe tricuspid regurgitation had widening of LV and RV diastolic pressures and accentuation of the

$$SAI = \frac{RV\ area\ during\ inspiration/LV\ area\ during\ inspiration}{RV\ area\ during\ expiration/LV\ area\ during\ expiration}$$

In this analysis, an SAI ratio of greater than 1.1 had 97% sensitivity and 100% predictive accuracy for identifying patients with surgically proven constrictive pericarditis. Other findings that

height and slope of RV early rapid filling wave (**Fig. 7**). These findings occur more commonly in patients with tricuspid regurgitation because flow into the RV is not limited by the rigid pericardium

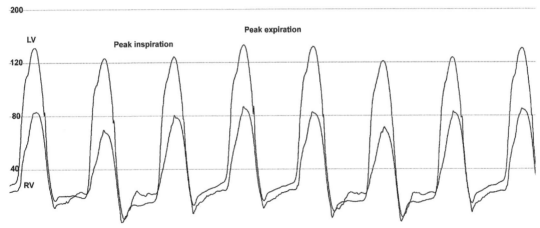

Fig. 4. Pressure recordings from a patient with restrictive cardiomyopathy. The LV and RV pressures move concordantly with respiration.

evident in patients with constrictive pericarditis. Thus, patients with tricuspid regurgitation have significant enhancement of RV diastolic filling during inspiration with a marked increase in RV diastolic pressures and rapid flow waves.

Other entities that may cause diastolic equalization include severe decompensated left-sided heart failure, severe tricuspid incompetence, RV dilatation from infarction, and acute mitral regurgitation secondary to rupture of the chordae tendinae. Of note, diastolic equalization may not be present in a patient with constrictive pericarditis with low to normal right atrial pressures from diuresis. Such patients demonstrate low cardiac output, and fluid challenge (>1 L saline bolus) is necessary to unmask the hemodynamic findings of constrictive pericarditis.[10]

CARDIAC TAMPONADE

Cardiac tamponade occurs when intrapericardial pressure exceeds intracardiac pressure, resulting in impairment of ventricular filling throughout the entire diastolic period. Virtually any disorder that causes pericardial effusion can result in cardiac tamponade. The most common cause is malignancy, with breast and lung cancer being the most frequent. Other important causes are complications of invasive cardiac procedures, idiopathic or viral pericarditis, aortic dissection with disruption of the aortic valve annulus, tuberculosis, uremia, and pericarditis or ventricular wall rupture from myocardial infarction.

Echocardiography is the primary modality for diagnosing cardiac tamponade. However, the increasing complexity of invasive cardiac procedures and their potential association with tamponade necessitates familiarity with the

manifestations and treatment of tamponade in the catheterization laboratory.

Pathophysiology

The pericardium normally contains 15 to 50 mL of fluid between the parietal and visceral layers, with intrapericardial pressure approximating intrapleural pressure (-5 to $+5$ cm H_2O). The amount and rate of fluid accumulation determine the hemodynamic effects of a pericardial effusion.[11,12] Intrapericardial pressure increases with fluid accumulation and pericardial restraint. Venous return and ventricular filling become impaired once the intrapericardial pressure exceeds the filling pressure of the cardiac chambers. This impairment precipitates a reduction in cardiac output, followed by increases in pulmonary venous and jugular venous pressures. With inspiration, there is a reduction in the driving pressure to fill the LV, subsequently leading to a reduction in ventricular filling and stroke volume. The reduction in LV stroke volume during inspiration manifests as a relative decrease in pulse pressure or peak systolic pressure, which is the hallmark finding of pulsus paradoxus in patients with cardiac tamponade.

There are uncommon clinical presentations of cardiac tamponade. Cardiac tamponade may be localized when a loculated pericardial effusion is tactically located to impair ventricular filling. This manifestation may occur in the after cardiac surgery or other postoperative settings. The loculated effusion may be present in the posterior pericardial space adjacent to the atria, which poses challenges for detection by echocardiography. Posterior loculated effusion should be suspected in postoperative patient with hemodynamic instability.

A

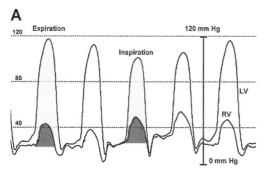

B

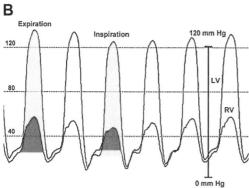

Fig. 5. The SAI for differentiating constrictive pericarditis from restrictive cardiomyopathy. These are high-fidelity micromanometer pressure tracings from 2 patients during inspiration and expiration. In both patients, there is early rapid ventricular filling and diastolic equalization at end expiration. (*A*) In a patient with constrictive pericarditis, there is an increase in the area of the RV pressure curve (*orange shaded area*) during inspiration compared with expiration. The area of the LV pressure curve (*yellow shaded area*) decreases during inspiration as compared with expiration. (*B*) Conversely, in a patient with restrictive cardiomyopathy, there is a decrease in the area of the RV pressure curve (*orange shaded area*) as compared with expiration. The area of the LV pressure curve (*yellow shaded area*) is unchanged during inspiration as compared with expiration. (*Reprinted from* Talreja DR, Nishimura RA, Oh JK, et al. Constrictive pericarditis in the modern era: novel criteria for diagnosis in the cardiac catheterization laboratory. J Am Coll Cardiol 2008;51:315–9; with permission.)

Low-pressure tamponade occurs without elevated jugular venous pressure because the intracardiac filling pressures are low.[13] Examples of this manifestation are patients with tuberculosis or malignancy complicated by severe dehydration. Finally, pneumopericardium with cardiac tamponade may result from gas-forming bacterial pericarditis after penetrating chest trauma.

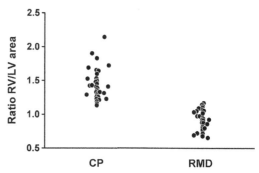

Fig. 6. Utility of the SAI for differentiating constrictive pericarditis from restrictive cardiomyopathy. A scatter plot of the ratio of RV to LV area during expiration versus inspiration. CP, constrictive pericarditis; RMD, restrictive cardiomyopathy. (*Reprinted from* Talreja DR, Nishimura RA, Oh JK, et al. Constrictive pericarditis in the modern era: novel criteria for diagnosis in the cardiac catheterization laboratory. J Am Coll Cardiol 2008;51:315–9; with permission.)

Diagnosis

Cardiac tamponade should be suspected when there is a compatible history, hypotension, and an elevated jugular venous pressure or pulsus paradoxus. The chest radiograph (eg, water-bottle heart) and electrocardiography (ECG, eg, sinus tachycardia, electrical alternans) may be helpful. However, the primary test for confirmation of the diagnosis is echocardiography.

Two-dimensional echocardiography readily detects pericardial effusions. Signs of cardiac tamponade include collapse of the right atrium and RV, ventricular septal shifting with respiration, and enlargement of the inferior vena cava.[14] With Doppler echocardiography, respiratory variation in mitral inflow can be detected early in the evolution of tamponade.[15] Moreover, the changes in mitral inflow are highly sensitive and may precede changes in cardiac output, blood pressure, and other echocardiographic evidence of tamponade. Respiratory changes in mitral inflow resolve after pericardiocentesis unless effusive-constrictive physiology is present.

Invasive Hemodynamics

Cardiac catheterization is usually not needed to make the diagnosis of cardiac tamponade. In these patients, the atrial pressure tracing typically is elevated, with prominent *x* descents and blunted or absent *y* descents (**Fig. 8**). Preservation of the *x* descent occurs because systolic ejection leads to a decrease in intracardiac volume and a temporary reduction in right atrial and intrapericardial

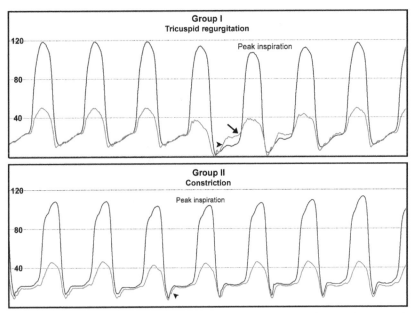

Fig. 7. Hemodynamic findings of constrictive pericarditis versus severe tricuspid regurgitation. Enhanced ventricular interdependence may be present in both disorders. In a patient with severe tricuspid regurgitation (*top*), deep inspiration leads to separation of the diastolic pressures with a higher RV diastolic pressure (*arrowhead*), and the rapid filling wave in the RV (*arrow*) becomes deeper and steeper. In the patient with constrictive pericarditis (*bottom*), there is elevation and equalization of diastolic pressures. However, the RV rapid filling wave (*arrowhead*) is not accentuated on inspiration. (*Reprinted from* Jaber WA, Sorajja P, Borlaug BA, et al. Differentiation of tricuspid regurgitation from constrictive pericarditis: novel criteria for diagnosis in the cardiac catheterization laboratory. Heart 2009;95:1449–54; with permission.)

pressures. During the remainder of the cardiac cycle, elevated intrapericardial pressure impairs ventricular filling, leading to blunting or obliteration of the *y* descent. Corresponding changes are also seen in ventricular pressure tracings with elevated diastolic pressures and loss or blunting of early diastolic pressure (or ventricular minimum pressure). Other hemodynamic findings include equalization of end-diastolic pressures, reduced cardiac output, and alterations in the systolic ejection period or pulse pressure that result from decreased stroke volume and are analogous to the bedside finding of pulsus paradoxus. During pericardiocentesis, intrapericardial pressure is elevated and should be equal to the intracardiac end-diastolic pressure.

Pericardiocentesis

Historically, pericardiocentesis was performed in a blinded or ECG-guided fashion, usually from the subxyphoid approach. Although these techniques may still be useful in some situations (eg, emergencies or cardiogenic shock), the incidence of complications is high, and echocardiographic guidance is strongly preferred.[16] Of note, care

should be taken to avoid pericardiocentesis in the treatment of tamponade that occurs with aortic dissection. In these patients, abrupt return of ventricular ejection may exacerbate the dissection and precipitate acute decompensation in these patients.[17]

- Echocardiography is used to determine the most appropriate portal of entry and needle direction into the pericardial effusion. The window closest to the effusion is usually selected. The most commonly used site is apical, but locations that have been used are axillary, left or right parasternal, and the subxyphoid window. With the imaging probe in place, the needle trajectory should be predetermined by the operator. Care should be taken to avoid the internal mammary or intercostal arteries. The entry site can be marked with an indelible pen.
- Local anesthesia is administered.
- Using the predetermined angulation, a polytef-sheathed needle is inserted at the entry site and advanced with gentle aspiration into the pericardial space. Once fluid is obtained, the needle is advanced slightly

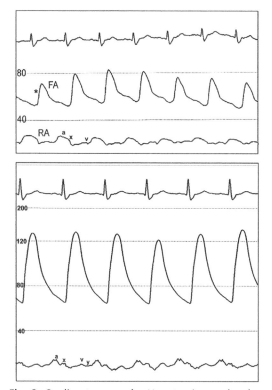

Fig. 8. Cardiac tamponade. Hypotension and pulsus paradoxus (*asterisk*) in the femoral artery (FA) pressure tracing and loss of the *y* descent in the right atrial (RA) pressure tracing is evident (*top*). After pericardiocentesis, there is an increase in arterial pressure and return of the *y* descent in RA pressure tracing (*bottom*).

further (approximately 2–3 mm) to completely place the polytef sheath in the pericardial space. The polytef sheath then is advanced over the needle, followed by withdrawal of the needle. The needle should not be readvanced into the sheath once it has been removed.

- Agitated saline is injected into the polytef sheath via a 3-way stopcock under echocardiography. If contrast does not opacify the pericardial space, then the catheter should be repositioned by withdrawal or passage of another needle and sheath. As noted previously, the needle should not be advanced back into the sheath once it has been removed.
- Once the intrapericardial position of the polytef sheath is confirmed, it is exchanged over a standard guidewire for a 5 or 6 Fr introducer sheath, followed by placement of a multilumen pigtail catheter in the pericardial space. The introducer sheath subsequently is removed, leaving only the

smooth walled pigtail catheter in place. If needed, reconfirmation of the catheter location with measurement of intrapericardial pressure and saline injection can be performed.

- The pericardial effusion is removed using either vacuum bottle or manual techniques with removal as much as possible to promote reapposition of the parietal and visceral pericardial surfaces. This apposition promotes adhesions that prevent fluid recurrence. Echocardiography is used to monitor fluid removal. If drainage stops despite residual effusion on echocardiography, the pigtail should be repositioned.
- The pigtail catheter is aspirated every 4 to 6 hours and flushed with heparinized saline. The catheter can be removed when the drainage is minimal (<25 mL per 24 hours), and repeat echocardiography reveals no significant residual effusion.

Occasionally, the tense pericardium may discharge fluid from the pericardial effusion into the pleural space during attempts at needle passage. This effect can be immediately recognized on echocardiography and may obviate further attempts at pericardiocentesis because acute relief from tamponade may occur. Although the vast majority of pericardial effusions can be treated percutaneously, some still require subxyphoid surgical drainage. Surgical approach may be required for viscous or loculated effusions or those resulting from bacterial infections. Recent hemorrhage into the pericardium also may result in pericardial clot formation that can be difficult to remove with a catheter. The true posterior effusion may be difficult to approach from any thoracic window and may require surgery.

KEY POINTS

1. Early rapid ventricular filling (ie, dip and plateau pattern) can be seen in patients with constrictive pericarditis, restrictive cardiomyopathy, or any volume overload state that results in pericardial restraint. Underdamping of fluid-filled catheters may mimic this pattern of ventricular filling.
2. Both traditional and dynamic respiratory criteria should be used to distinguish constrictive pericarditis from restrictive cardiomyopathy. Dynamic respiratory criteria for constrictive pericarditis are (1) discordance of the RV and LV systolic pressures due to enhanced ventricular interdependence; and (2) dissociation of intrathoracic and intracavitary pressures.

3. The hemodynamic hallmarks of cardiac tamponade are pulsus paradoxus and loss of the *y* descent in the atrial waveform. Blunting of early ventricular filling also may occur.

REFERENCES

1. McCaughan BC, Schaff HV, Piehler JM, et al. Early and late results of pericardiectomy for constrictive pericarditis. J Thorac Cardiovasc Surg 1985;89:340–50.
2. Ammash NM, Seward JB, Bailey KR, et al. Clinical profile and outcome of idiopathic restrictive cardiomyopathy. Circulation 2000;101:2490–6.
3. Arbustini E, Morbini P, Grasso M, et al. Restrictive cardiomyopathy, atrioventricular block and mild to subclinical myopathy in patients with desmin–immunoreactive material deposits. J Am Coll Cardiol 1998;31:645–53.
4. Zhang J, Kumar A, Stalker HJ, et al. Clinical and molecular studies of a large family with desmin–associated restrictive cardiomyopathy. Clin Genet 2001;59:248–56.
5. Mogensen J, Kubo T, Duque M, et al. Idiopathic restrictive cardiomyopathy is part of the clinical expression of cardiac troponin I mutations. J Clin Invest 2003;111:209–16.
6. Lorell BH, Grossman W. Profiles in constrictive pericarditis, restrictive cardiomyopathy, and cardiac–tamponade. In: Grossman W, editor. Cardiac catheterization and angiography. Philadelphia: Lea & Febiger; 1986. p. 427–45.
7. Hurrell DG, Nishimura RA, Higano ST, et al. Value of dynamic respiratory changes in left and right ventricular pressures for the diagnosis of constrictive pericarditis. Circulation 1996;93:2007–13.
8. Talreja DR, Nishimura RA, Oh JK, et al. Constrictive pericarditis in the modern era: novel criteria for diagnosis in the cardiac catheterization laboratory. J Am Coll Cardiol 2008;51:315–9.
9. Jaber WA, Sorajja P, Borlaug BA, et al. Differentiation of tricuspid regurgitation from constrictive pericarditis: novel criteria for diagnosis in the cardiac catheterization laboratory. Heart 2009;95:1449–54.
10. Bush CA, Stang JM, Wooley CF, et al. Occult constrictive pericardial disease. Diagnosis by rapid volume expansion and correction by pericardiectomy. Circulation 1977;56:924–30.
11. Spodick DH. Acute cardiac tamponade. N Engl J Med 2003;349:684–90.
12. Shabetai R. The pathophysiology of cardiac tamponade. Cardiovasc Clin 1976;7:67–89.
13. Antman EM, Cargill V, Grossman W. Low–pressure cardiac tamponade. Ann Intern Med 1979;91:403–6.
14. Armstrong WF, Schilt BF, Helper DJ, et al. Diastolic collapse of the right ventricle with cardiac tamponade: an echocardiographic study. Circulation 1982;65:1491–6.
15. Burstow DJ, Oh JK, Bailey KR, et al. Cardiac tamponade: characteristic Doppler observations. Mayo Clin Proc 1989;64:312–24.
16. Tsang TS, Freeman WK, Sinak LJ, et al. Echocardiographically guided pericardiocentesis: evolution and state-of-the-art technique. Mayo Clin Proc 1998;73:647–52.
17. Isselbacher EM, Cigarroa JE, Eagle KA. Cardiac tamponade complicating proximal aortic dissection. Is pericardiocentesis harmful? Circulation 1994;90:2375–8.

Contemporary Application of Cardiovascular Hemodynamics: Transcatheter Mitral Valve Interventions

Hasan Jilaihawi, MD, Raj Makkar, MD,
Asma Hussaini, MS, PA-C, Alfredo Trento, MD,
Saibal Kar, MD*

KEYWORDS
• Mitral regurgitation • Mitral stenosis • Hemodynamics
• Mitral valvuloplasty • PTMV • MitraClip

The mainstay for the hemodynamic assessment of the mitral valve has, for some time, been echocardiography, and this modality continues to evolve with the advent and refinement of 3-dimensional (3D) transesophageal technologies.[1] The American College of Cardiology/American Heart Association guidelines state that today transcatheter "hemodynamic measurements are indicated when there is a discrepancy between clinical and noninvasive findings regarding severity of MR."[2] However, such a discrepancy may not be infrequent; the best echocardiographic tools for distinguishing severe from nonsevere mitral regurgitation (MR) are only modestly reliable and associated with suboptimal interobserver agreement.[3] Thus, the need for an understanding of transcatheter hemodynamics may extend beyond the catheterization laboratory to both imaging and general cardiologists, as well as to the surgeons to whom patients with mitral valve disease are referred.

Although the transcatheter assessment of mitral valve hemodynamics has remained pivotal in the periprocedural guidance of percutaneous transluminal mitral valvuloplasty (PTMV) and in the assessment of its efficacy and potential complications,[4] the decline in the incidence of rheumatic mitral valve disease[5] has meant that the skills in their interpretation are maintained only by a select few involved with this increasingly rare procedure.

In recent years, there has been considerable preliminary success in the novel therapy for transcatheter mitral valve repair for MR using MitraClip (Abbott Vascular, Santa Clara, CA, USA),[6,7] a pathologic condition that continues to increase in prevalence.[8] Pivotal to the optimal performance of this procedure is the symbiotic interpretation in real time of advanced ultrasound-based imaging and precise transcatheter hemodynamic interpretation, accompanied only by limited x-ray fluoroscopy. This article discusses and illustrates the key components of the hemodynamic assessment of mitral valve disease through the established PTMV for rheumatic mitral stenosis and the novel MitraClip repair for nonrheumatic MR.

Cedars-Sinai Heart Institute, Cedars-Sinai Medical Center, 8700 Beverly Boulevard, Los Angeles, CA 90048, USA
* Corresponding author.
E-mail address: karsk@cshs.org

Cardiol Clin 29 (2011) 201–209
doi:10.1016/j.ccl.2011.01.005
0733-8651/11/$ – see front matter © 2011 Elsevier Inc. All rights reserved.

KEY COMPONENTS OF THE HEMODYNAMIC ASSESSMENT OF MITRAL INTERVENTIONS

The following are the critical invasive parameters that should be scrutinized systematically in the assessment of mitral valve physiology:

1. The left atrial (LA) pressure (or pulmonary capillary wedge pressure [PCWP]), both the mean pressure and waveform morphology, with particular emphasis on the v wave.

The v wave is perhaps the most dynamic indicator in transcatheter mitral valve intervention. It occurs during ventricular systole and indicates LA filling, which may be antegrade from the pulmonary veins or retrograde from the left ventricle (LV). This wave is prominent in severe mitral stenosis (**Fig. 1**), in which it indicates accelerated antegrade passive filling associated with noncompliance of the LA. In severe MR, the v wave indicates a regurgitant jet commencing before ventricular systole.

Although the PCWP is a reliable surrogate for LA pressure, both dampened and inaccurately high waveforms have been reported (**Fig. 2**),[9] which means that direct LA pressure evaluation is preferable[10] and is always available in transcatheter mitral interventions. The v-wave height itself is a poor measure of MR severity.[9] The size of the v wave is determined by the timing of LA filling in relation to the LA compliance curve period rather than the degree of filling per se.[11] In line with this fact, besides mitral stenosis and MR, other diseases that increase volume or flow in a noncompliant LA, such as ventricular septal defects, can also produce large v waves.[11] Rather than the absolute reading of the v wave it is the trend from its baseline reading that is of greatest value.

The mean LA pressure itself, although useful, is a less-reliable indicator of mitral valve physiology.[12] It may be overestimated or underestimated by the PCWP (see **Fig. 2**).[9] Failure of LA pressure to come down in PTMV may indicate a failure to relieve stenosis or an iatrogenic MR.

The LA pressure may be normal even in the setting of severe MR[12] and may remain normal until advanced stages of decompensation. The LA pressure can be low in severe MR in the setting of hypotension or during anesthesia, as well as in chronic compensated MR. In MR, the LA pressure may have diurnal variation and vary with activity. The authors have observed an immediate reduction in LA pressure even in severe functional MR after MitraClip therapy (**Fig. 3**).

2. The mean transmitral gradient between the mean LA pressure and the LV end-diastolic pressure.

It is important to appreciate that the gradient may be influenced both by obstruction and increased flow, as in significant MR. Although mitral valve gradients can be completely eliminated by balloon valvuloplasty, the gradient reduction may be modest or absent if significant regurgitation ensues as a complication.[13] In atrial fibrillation, because of a beat-to-beat variation in stroke volume, mitral valve gradient measurements should be averaged over 10 consecutive beats (5 in sinus rhythm).[14]

3. The cardiac output (CO) should ideally be calculated before and after a mitral intervention and is rapidly assessed by the thermodilution method. An important caveat is that this method is not reliable in the presence of coexisting shunting, which could be the case after a transseptal puncture, in which the more time-consuming Fick method has to be used[15]; the presence of a significant shunt can be determined by periprocedural transesophageal echocardiogram (TEE). Thus, assessment of CO after transcatheter mitral procedures, such as PTMV and MitraClip therapy, should be done before the catheter is removed from across the interatrial septum.

A drop in CO after PTMV may indicate new significant MR. Effective (forward) CO is usually depressed in symptomatic MR, whereas total LV output is usually elevated. CO during exercise is the main determinant of the functional status in MR. A failure of the CO to increase after transcatheter mitral repair by MitraClip may indicate hemodynamically significant residual MR.

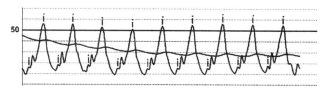

Fig. 1. The v wave is prominent in severe mitral stenosis, indicating accelerated antegrade passive filling associated with noncompliance of the LA.

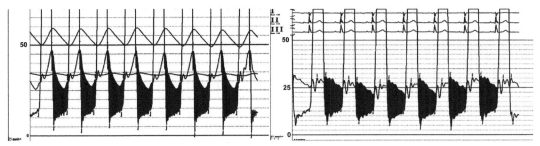

Fig. 2. Disparity between direct LA pressure measurement and PCWP estimation.

4. When available, the TEE, which should always be regarded as providing complementary data to catheter-derived data, should be used.

TEE is useful in PTMV for the evaluation of safety and efficacy, in the transseptal puncture, in the evaluation of reduction of mitral gradient by commissurotomy, and the avoidance of severe MR and provides data that complement those derived from transcatheter hemodynamics. However, TEE is essential in the MitraClip procedure and should ideally use a 3D system. TEE guides positioning in real time, assesses improvement in MR directly and by resolution of pulmonary vein flow reversal (the echocardiographic parallel of v-wave reduction), and evaluates the safety of a second clip when deployed using gradients (whereby a mean of 2–4 mm Hg is satisfactory) and double-orifice planimetry (mitral valve area >2 cm²).

TRANSCATHETER HEMODYNAMICS AND PTMV

PTMV is an effective treatment of rheumatic mitral stenosis.[16] Its basis is the principle of a controlled commissural tear, relieving stenosis but not disrupting the function of the mitral valve or its subvalvular apparatus to the level at which significant insufficiency ensues. Pivotal to the success of this procedure is the symbiotic interpretation in real time of data from fluoroscopy, precise transcatheter hemodynamic interpretation, and, preferably, intraprocedural ultrasound-based imaging.

When performed optimally, there is a reduction in the v wave, mean LA pressure, and transmitral gradient (**Fig. 4**) and an increase in CO.

Echocardiography, performed intraprocedurally or periprocedurally, provides further confirmation of optimal mitral valve hemodynamics. Echocardiographically, severe mitral stenosis is defined as a mean gradient greater than 10 mm Hg and a valve area less than 1 cm².[2] Historically, procedural success has been defined arbitrarily as an adequate valve area by Gorlin calculation, echocardiographic planimetry, or Doppler (≥1.5 cm²), with an increase of 25% or more in the absence of significant (≥2+ ie, moderate or severe) MR.[17] Harcombe and colleagues[4] found the Gorlin method of mitral valve area calculation to be a more heart rate–independent measure than Doppler after valvuloplasty.

There is some recent prognostic evidence that a higher cutoff for valve area of 1.8 cm² or more should be used in the definition of procedural success based on the likelihood of subsequent long-term restenosis.[18] Anatomic case selection has been well validated for procedural safety using the Massachusetts General Hospital (MGH) score

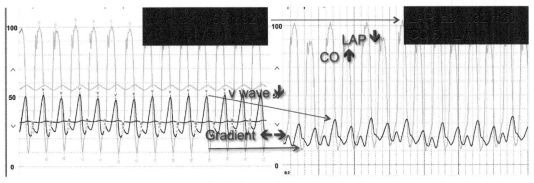

Fig. 3. Immediate reduction in LA pressure (LAP) observed after MitraClip therapy in severe functional MR, with an accompanying increase in cardiac output (CO). a, peak "a wave" pressure; m, mean LAP; v, peak "v wave" pressure; ↑, increases; ↓, decreases; ← →, remains the same.

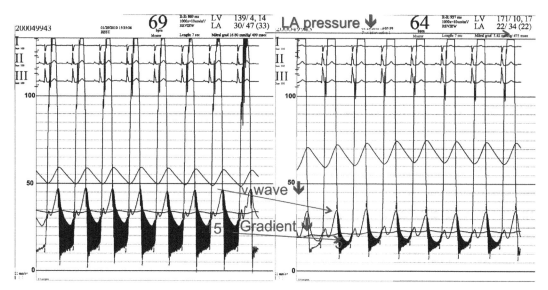

Fig. 4. An optimal hemodynamic outcome after PTMV with a reduction in the v wave, mean LA pressure, and transmitral gradient. ↑, increases; ↓, decreases; ← →, remains the same.

of 8 or less.[19] The Inoue balloon (Toray Industries Inc, Tokyo, Japan) is most widely used, with a stepwise dilatation technique, using transcatheter and echocardiographic assessments before a gradual 0.5- to 1-mL further increase in balloon volume for dilatation[20]; the starting balloon volume can be estimated by the formula (patient height in centimeters/10)+10 milliliters.[21]

A suboptimal result with an increase in MR and residual mitral stenosis can be detected with transcatheter hemodynamics and confirmed by echocardiography. An increase in the v wave, a residual gradient caused both by some residual stenosis and the increased flow associated with MR, and a slight increase in LA pressure may be seen (**Fig. 5**). There may be an accompanying reduction in CO.

Despite a stepwise technique, PTMV may, on rare occasions, result in catastrophic MR, with an accompanying dramatic increase in the v

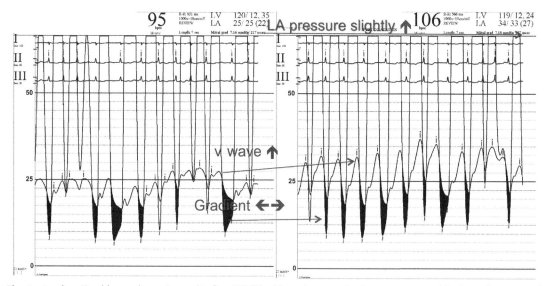

Fig. 5. A suboptimal hemodynamic result after PTMV with an increase in the v wave, a residual gradient caused both by some residual stenosis and an increased flow associated with MR, and a slight increase in LA pressure. Echocardiography confirmed mild residual mitral stenosis with new moderate regurgitation. ↑, increases; ↓, decreases; ← →, remains the same.

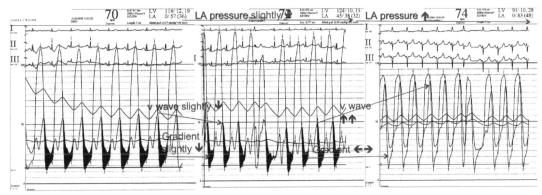

Fig. 6. Catastrophic MR after PTMV, with an accompanying dramatic increase in the v wave and LA pressure and the gradient of mitral stenosis being replaced by a gradient of increased flow because of MR. This patient was stabilized emergently with an intra-aortic balloon pump and had a favorable outcome after mitral valve replacement. ↑, increases; ↓, decreases; ← →, remains the same.

wave and LA pressure and the gradient of mitral stenosis being replaced by a gradient of increased flow because of MR (**Fig. 6**). In addition to the MGH score, the presence of excessive commissural calcification is an important adverse risk factor for such a complication. Because PTMV relies on the principle of commissural separation along the path of least resistance, the presence of commissural calcification means that this path becomes leaflets rather than commissures, which is when catastrophic leaflet tears and severe MR may ensue. This gradient is driven by increased flow rather than stenosis and has a characteristically more V-shaped morphology with a steeper

upstroke of the LV diastolic waveform; this is not seen if severe stenosis remains as diastolic LV filling is impaired.

TRANSCATHETER HEMODYNAMICS AND PERCUTANEOUS MITRAL VALVE REPAIR USING THE MITRACLIP

MitraClip percutaneous mitral valve repair (PMVR) is effective in nonrheumatic MR, in which an incompetent single-orifice valve is converted to a competent double-orifice valve, inevitably decreasing the mitral valve area to some extent.[22] For this reason, the baseline mitral valve area must be greater than

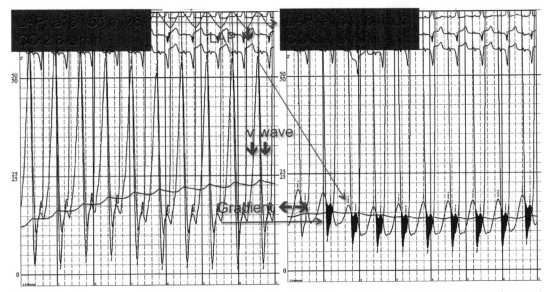

Fig. 7. Optimal outcome after 2-clip PMVR, with significant MR attenuated dramatically to only trivial regurgitation; a dramatic reduction in the v wave is seen, with LA pressure (LAP) reduced or unchanged, no increase in transmitral gradient, and an increase in CO. a, peak "a wave" pressure; m, mean LAP; v, peak "v wave" pressure; ↑, increases; ↓, decreases; ← →, remains the same.

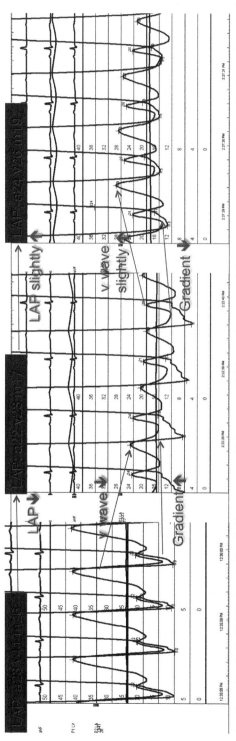

Fig. 8. Obstruction after 2-clip PMVR. A reduction in the v wave and LA pressure (LAP) may be seen and demonstrate amelioration of MR, but hemodynamically important obstruction was indicated by a significant increase in transmitral gradient in this case. The second clip was removed, accepting some residual MR. a, peak "a wave" pressure; m, mean LAP; v, peak "v wave" pressure; ↑, increases; ↓, decreases; ← →, remains the same.

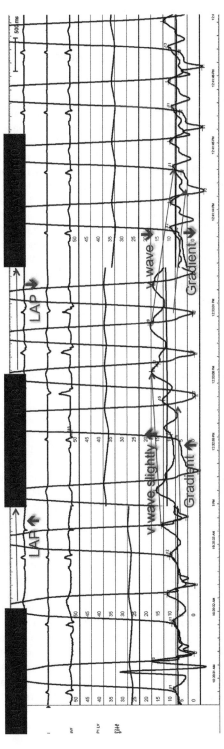

Fig. 9. Suboptimal hemodynamic outcome after single-clip PMVR, optimized with a second clip. The first clip failed to improve the severe MR but caused a mild stenosis and an increase in transmitral gradient. The rapid upstroke of the LV waveform in late diastole indicates an increased flow in the absence of major obstruction, and hence predominant regurgitation. Paradoxically, a second clip, reduced the MR without aggravating obstruction. This amelioration of MR relieved the gradient, with an accompanying reduction in the v wave and LA pressure (LAP). a, peak "a wave" pressure; m, mean LAP; v, peak "v wave" pressure; ↑, increases; ↓, decreases; ←→, remains the same.

or equal to 4 cm^2. This technique is effective in selected patients with functional or degenerative MR.

The acute hemodynamics after mitral valve surgery are confounded by an acute postoperative low output state, related in part to cardioplegia. This is not the case after PMVR, which is influenced purely by MR reduction. Pivotal to the optimal performance of this procedure is the symbiotic interpretation in real time of advanced ultrasound-based imaging and precise transcatheter hemodynamic interpretation, supported by only limited x-ray fluoroscopy.

In optimal MitraClip PMVR, significant MR is attenuated dramatically to mild MR or MR of less severity using 1 or 2 clips. A dramatic reduction in the v wave is seen, with a decrease or no change in the LA pressure, no significant increase in transmitral gradient, and an increase in the CO (**Fig. 7**). Although a visual qualitative assessment and resolution of pulmonary vein flow reversal may be of value, the echocardiographic assessment of residual MR with a double-orifice mitral valve is not well understood and double proximal isovelocity surface area and vena contracta methodologies are most probably invalid in this setting. The above-mentioned shortfalls make transcatheter hemodynamic assessment of great importance, of particular value being the v wave amelioration. This should arguably be incorporated into the definition of procedural success.

When a second clip is necessary, it must be ensured that the benefit of a further reduction in MR is not offset by an increase in obstruction. Although a reduction in the v wave and LA pressure may be seen and demonstrate amelioration of MR, hemodynamically important obstruction is indicated by a significant increase in transmitral gradient (**Fig. 8**). In this setting, the second clip can be easily removed, accepting some residual MR.

In contrast, an increase in gradient with Mitra-Clip PMVR does not always indicate predominant obstruction. If the first clip fails to ameliorate MR but causes a mild stenosis, a gradient can arise, but the rapid upstroke of the LV waveform in late diastole indicates increased flow in the absence of major obstruction and hence predominant regurgitation (**Fig. 9**). Paradoxically, a second clip, by reducing the MR without aggravating obstruction, can relieve this gradient, with an accompanying reduction in the v wave and LA pressure.

SUMMARY

Catheter-based hemodynamics is of critical importance during percutaneous mitral valve interventions. Changes in the LA pressure and waveform, mean gradient, and CO are important assessment parameters for both safety and efficacy. Invasive hemodynamics is complementary to echocardiographic imaging in this setting.

REFERENCES

1. Macnab A, Jenkins NP, Bridgewater BJ, et al. Three-dimensional echocardiography is superior to multiplane transoesophageal echo in the assessment of regurgitant mitral valve morphology. Eur J Echocardiogr 2004;5:212–22.

2. Bonow RO, Carabello BA, Chatterjee K, et al. 2008 Focused update incorporated into the ACC/AHA 2006 guidelines for the management of patients with valvular heart disease: a report of the American College of Cardiology/American Heart Association Task Force on Practice Guidelines (Writing Committee to revise the 1998 guidelines for the management of patients with valvular heart disease). Endorsed by the Society of Cardiovascular Anesthesiologists, Society for Cardiovascular Angiography and Interventions, and Society of Thoracic Surgeons. J Am Coll Cardiol 2008;52:e1–142.

3. Biner S, Rafique A, Rafii F, et al. Reproducibility of proximal isovelocity surface area, vena contracta, and regurgitant jet area for assessment of mitral regurgitation severity. JACC Cardiovasc Imaging 2010;3:235–43.

4. Harcombe AA, Ludman PF, Wisbey C, et al. Balloon mitral valvuloplasty: comparison of haemodynamic and echocardiographic assessment of mitral stenosis at different heart rates in the catheterisation laboratory. Int J Cardiol 1999;68:253–9.

5. Chandrashekhar Y, Westaby S, Narula J. Mitral stenosis. Lancet 2009;374:1271–83.

6. Feldman T, Kar S, Rinaldi M, et al. Percutaneous mitral repair with the MitraClip system: safety and midterm durability in the initial EVEREST (Endovascular Valve Edge-to-Edge REpair Study) cohort. J Am Coll Cardiol 2009;54:686–94.

7. Tamburino C, Ussia GP, Maisano F, et al. Percutaneous mitral valve repair with the MitraClip system: acute results from a real world setting. Eur Heart J 2010;31:1382–9.

8. Enriquez-Sarano M, Akins CW, Vahanian A. Mitral regurgitation. Lancet 2009;373:1382–94.

9. Freihage JH, Joyal D, Arab D, et al. Invasive assessment of mitral regurgitation: comparison of hemodynamic parameters. Catheter Cardiovasc Interv 2007;69:303–12.

10. Kern MJ. Hemodynamic rounds series II: mitral stenosis and pulsus alternans. Cathet Cardiovasc Diagn 1998;43:313–7.

11. Kern MJ, Deligonul U. Interpretation of cardiac pathophysiology from pressure waveform analysis: the

left-sided V wave. Cathet Cardiovasc Diagn 1991; 23:211–8.

12. Braunwald E, Awe WC. The syndrome of severe mitral regurgitation with normal left atrial pressure. Circulation 1963;27:29–35.

13. Kern MJ, Aguirre FV. Interpretation of cardiac pathophysiology from pressure waveform analysis: mitral valve gradients: part II. Cathet Cardiovasc Diagn 1992;27:52–6.

14. Kern MJ, Aguirre F. Interpretation of cardiac pathophysiology from pressure waveform analysis: mitral valve gradients: part I. Cathet Cardiovasc Diagn 1992;26:308–15.

15. Wilkinson JL. Haemodynamic calculations in the catheter laboratory. Heart 2001;85:113–20.

16. Vahanian A, Palacios IF. Percutaneous approaches to valvular disease. Circulation 2004;109:1572–9.

17. Abascal VM, Wilkins GT, O'Shea JP, et al. Prediction of successful outcome in 130 patients undergoing percutaneous balloon mitral valvotomy. Circulation 1990;82:448–56.

18. Song JK, Song JM, Kang DH, et al. Restenosis and adverse clinical events after successful percutaneous mitral valvuloplasty: immediate post-procedural mitral valve area as an important prognosticator. Eur Heart J 2009;30:1254–62.

19. Wilkins GT, Weyman AE, Abascal VM, et al. Percutaneous balloon dilatation of the mitral valve: an analysis of echocardiographic variables related to outcome and the mechanism of dilatation. Br Heart J 1988;60:299–308.

20. Inoue K, Owaki T, Nakamura T, et al. Clinical application of transvenous mitral commissurotomy by a new balloon catheter. J Thorac Cardiovasc Surg 1984;87: 394–402.

21. Sanchez PL, Harrell LC, Salas RE, et al. Learning curve of the Inoue technique of percutaneous mitral balloon valvuloplasty. Am J Cardiol 2001;88:662–7.

22. Herrmann HC, Kar S, Siegel R, et al. Effect of percutaneous mitral repair with the MitraClip device on mitral valve area and gradient. EuroIntervention 2009;4:437–42.

Contemporary Application of Cardiovascular Hemodynamics: Transcatheter Aortic Valve Interventions

Hasan Jilaihawi, MD, Saibal Kar, MD, Niraj Doctor, MD, Gregory Fontana, MD, Raj Makkar, MD*

KEYWORDS

- Transcatheter aortic valve implantation
- Percutaneous aortic valve replacement
- Edwards Sapien valve • Medtronic CoreValve
- Hemodynamics • Aortic stenosis

Over the past two decades, echocardiography has replaced cardiac catheterization for aortic valvular hemodynamic assessment. In recent years, however, there has been a rapid evolution of transcatheter aortic valve technology and, with its refinement, there has been the increasing recognition of the value of transcatheter hemodynamic assessment in complementing the information provided by contemporary echocardiography. With an emphasis on transcatheter hemodynamics, this article reviews the symbiotic application of these assessment modalities pertaining to contemporary transcatheter aortic valve implantation (TAVI).

FROM IN VITRO TO IN VIVO HEMODYNAMICS

Pulse duplicator and bioreactor models have been used for some time to assess the expected hemodynamic function of valvular prostheses.[1,2] In vitro assessment of balloon expandable Edwards Sapien transcatheter aortic valves (Edwards Lifesciences, Irvine, CA, USA) using such models (**Fig. 1**) suggests improved hemodynamics in relation to conventional aortic bioprostheses. Similar findings have been demonstrated in vivo, with favorable hemodynamics and a lower incidence of prosthesis-patient mismatch with the Edwards Sapien valve when compared with the surgical bioprostheses.[3] Equally favorable data have been established with the Medtronic CoreValve self-expanding transcatheter valve (Medtronic, Minneapolis, MN, USA).[4,5] Studies for both designs have documented that the optimal acute hemodynamics following TAVI for severe aortic stenosis (AS) (**Figs. 2** and **3**) are sustained at follow-up.[6,7]

PREOPERATIVE ASSESSMENT

It has long been known that the noninvasive assessment of AS with Doppler echocardiography generally corresponds well to that of invasive cardiac catheterization.[8–10] Provided noninvasive assessment is adequate and concordant with clinical findings, American College of Cardiology/American Heart Association (ACC/AHA) guidelines propose that transcatheter evaluation of AS carries a class III indication (not recommended).[11] Some

Cedars-Sinai Heart Institute, Cedars-Sinai Medical Center, 8700 Beverly Boulevard, Los Angeles, CA 90048, USA
* Corresponding author.
E-mail address: Raj.Makkar@cshs.org

Cardiol Clin 29 (2011) 211–222
doi:10.1016/j.ccl.2011.01.002

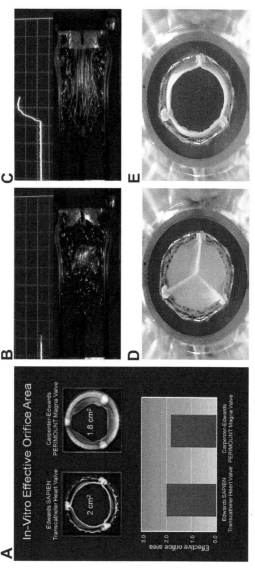

Fig. 1. In vitro transcatheter aortic valve hemodynamics. (*A*) The Edwards Sapien transcatheter aortic valve displays favorable in vitro hemodynamics when compared with the Edwards Perimount Magna conventional aortic valve (pulse duplicator data, Edwards Lifesciences). (*B, C*) Flow hemodynamics as seen with the model in cross section in diastole and systole, respectively. (*D, E*) Short-axis view of valve function in vitro, in diastole and systole, respectively.

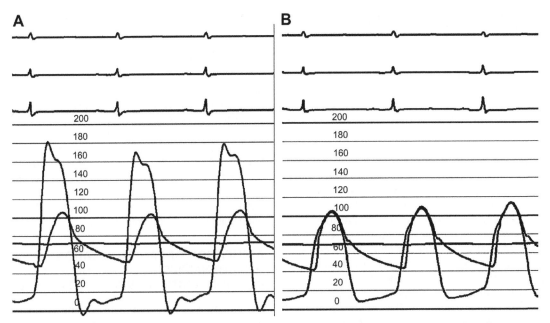

Fig. 2. Optimal hemodynamic waveforms post TAVI. Transaortic gradient resolved and diastolic pressure unchanged. (*A*) Pre-TAVI: severe aortic stenosis (AS), little or no aortic regurgitation (AR). (*B*) Post-TAVI: relief of AS, no AR.

commentators have lamented the decline in the understanding of cardiac catheterization hemodynamics,[12] which is all the more relevant in the era of transcatheter valve intervention. The contemporary value of a detailed preoperative transcatheter assessment is in the appreciation of the hemodynamics of an individual patient with a view to optimizing the ultimate TAVI procedure.

Either Doppler echocardiography or cardiac catheterization may be used for hemodynamic measurements with infusion of dobutamine, which can be useful for evaluation of patients with low-flow/low-gradient AS and left ventricular (LV) dysfunction; this carries a class IIa ACC/AHA indication.[11]

The transcatheter assessment of AS may be performed retrogradely by direct catheter

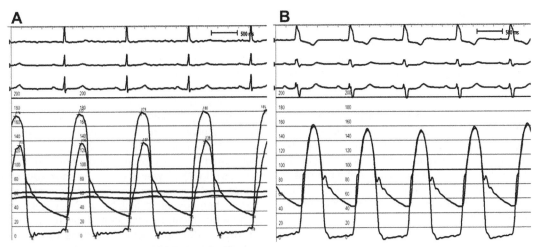

Fig. 3. Relief of mixed aortic valve disease by TAVI. (*A*) Severe AS is illustrated by the transaortic gradient and the slow upstroke of the systolic aortic waveform. Large pulse pressure and low diastolic pressure is indicative significant pre-TAVI AR. (*B*) Diastolic pressure increases after valve implantation, indicating relief of AR. Relief of AS is demonstrated not only by the improvement in gradient but also by the brisk upstroke of systolic waveform and recovery of a prominent dicrotic notch post procedure.

measurement either by a single-catheter or 2-catheter method. The single-catheter method can employ either pullback, which may be susceptible to errors relating to an increase in peripheral pressure, the so-called Carabello sign,[13] or use of the introducer side port (1F larger than the catheter) as a surrogate for aortic pressure; inaccuracies may arise given the difference in central aortic and femoral pressures. An alternative to the single-catheter method is the Langston dual-lumen catheter,[14] which provides a simultaneous measure of LV pressure and central aortic pressure; this requires special attention to the quality of the waveform, which may be dampened by the small-bore central lumen. A pressure wire assessment may minimize iatrogenic catheter-induced obstruction; the stenotic valve is crossed retrogradely with a catheter and straight wire, the pressure wire advanced through the catheter into the left ventricle, the catheter pulled back, and the gradient evaluated.[15] This relatively nonobstructive method can also be used for the evaluation of mechanical valves. An alternative to retrograde catheter assessment is a transseptal approach,[16] which is still frequently practiced in some centers worldwide; this avoids the possibility of iatrogenic dysfunction and valve-related emboli, but requires additional skills and carries a small risk of tamponade.

Severe septal hypertrophy can cause subvalvular AS that may coexist with valvular AS, and can be difficult to appreciate without a preoperative catheter assessment. This situation can be important during the procedure, with greater risk of embolization, and postprocedure, because despite TAVI the subvalvular stenosis may persist, which may cause the "suicide left ventricle" that is only unmasked after TAVI.[17] The hemodynamic waveform seen is the spike and dome similar to that seen in hypertrophic cardiomyopathy, with systolic anterior motion of the mitral valve. There is evidence for combined surgical septal myectomy and aortic valve replacement in this setting[18]; some operators have employed a lower than usual implantation position of the Edwards Sapien transcatheter valve[19] or the longer stent frame of the Medtronic CoreValve design[20,21] as transcatheter options. In any case, the presence of a prominent septal bulge on echocardiography should prompt a preoperative catheter assessment of the outflow tract gradient.

PERIPROCEDURAL APPLICATION OF HEMODYNAMIC PRINCIPLES

In all TAVI procedures, both echocardiography and transcatheter assessment can be used to provide valuable complementary information in real time. With the long stent frame of the self-expanding design, many operators employ a conscious sedation approach with no routine transesophageal echocardiography (TEE) guidance, and have complete reliance on intraprocedural fluoroscopically guided positioning and transcatheter hemodynamic evaluation. By contrast, with contemporary balloon-expandable TAVI, periprocedural TEE is mandatory, particularly in view of the precision of implantation dictated by the short stent frame; even in this setting, fluoroscopy and transcatheter evaluation, each with relative strengths, provide valuable and rapidly accessible information.

APPLICATION OF PREIMPLANTATION HEMODYNAMICS: RAPID PACING AND BALLOON AORTIC VALVULOPLASTY RESULTS

Hemodynamics are fundamental to the technique of TAVI with a beating-heart physiology. Rapid pacing at a heart rate of 180 to 220 beats per minute (bpm) facilitates the necessary depression in cardiac output, with a systolic arterial pressure of at least less than 60 mm Hg and a pulse pressure of less than 15 mm Hg,[22] to allow stable balloon inflation. This procedure is fundamental to predilatation and implantation of the balloon-expandable Edwards design and is preferred by many during the predilatation for the self-expanding Medtronic CoreValve design, in order to avoid excessive balloon movement. As an alternative to rapid pacing for predilatation with the self-expanding design, some operators advocate use of the Nucleus balloon (NuMED Canada Inc, Cornwall, ON, Canada), a dog-bone balloon that moves less during deflation. Rapid pacing is essential during any required postdilatation of both designs to avoid device embolization.

Although stand-alone balloon aortic valvuloplasty (BAV) is reemerging in the TAVI era,[23] it is a palliative or bridging therapy for patients with refractory symptoms, given the recoil phenomenon observed with calcific degenerative aortic valves.[24] Even in the acute setting, an optimally performed BAV can result in suboptimal hemodynamics (**Fig. 4**). However, overaggressive BAV can cause acute severe aortic regurgitation (AR) and further hemodynamic instability. Such instability can be dealt with by accelerated pacing at a rate of 100 to 120 bpm, which shortens diastole as a temporizing measure, allowing the procedure to be completed in a stable fashion (**Fig. 5**). This is a novel application of a long-established principle: relative tachycardia and reduction of AR is achieved by sublingual nifedipine,[25] which

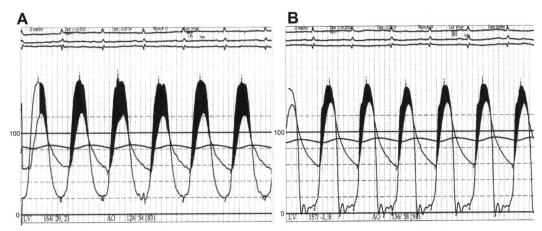

Fig. 4. Successful aortic valvuloplasty resulting in a suboptimal hemodynamic result. (*A*) Before BAV: mean gradient = 38 mm Hg with aortic valve area (AVA) = 0.48 cm². (*B*) After BAV: mean gradient = 26 mm Hg with AVA = 0.71 cm².

additionally exerts an effect through afterload reduction. Acute severe AR may result in severe dilatation of the left ventricle and refractory ventricular arrhythmia. If stability cannot be achieved, offloading the left ventricle with intra-procedural cardiopulmonary bypass may be necessary.

PERIPROCEDURAL ASSESSMENT OF AORTIC REGURGITATION

Paravalvular leak is always pathologic following conventional aortic valve surgery. However, a mild degree of paravalvular leak is a very common phenomenon following TAVI and is not associated with morbidity. Although only echocar-diography can reliably distinguish paravalvular leak from central leak during the procedure,

precise transcatheter hemodynamic assessment of AR is crucial to grading of its severity (**Figs. 6 and 7**), as the eccentricity of regurgitant jets can make the severity assessment by this modality extremely difficult. Moreover, aortography can yield unreliable data that are significantly affected by afterload, contrast volume, catheter height, and cardiac output.

An appreciation of transcatheter diastology is fundamental to the hemodynamic evaluation of post-TAVI AR. Postimplant hemodynamic data must be interpreted in the context of baseline diastolic parameters, which should be carefully documented. Diastolic dysfunction associated with LV hypertrophy may mean that even baseline end-diastolic pressure is elevated. However, a significant increase in end-diastolic pressure indicates important aortic insufficiency. An

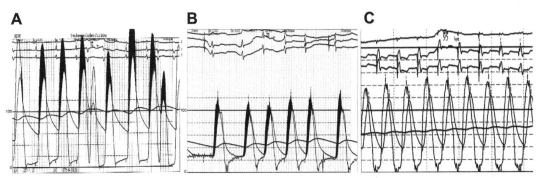

Fig. 5. Use of accelerated pacing to shorten diastole and reduce the hemodynamic impact of periprocedural severe AR. (*A*) Baseline. Aortic diastolic pressure 64 mm Hg, LV end-diastolic pressure (LVEDP) 16 mm Hg. (*B*) After balloon aortic valvuloplasty with aortic diastolic pressure 27 mm Hg ≈ LVEDP 24 mm Hg, that is, "diastasis." (*C*) Accelerated pacing at 90 to 100 bpm shortens diastole, increasing aortic diastolic pressure (42 mm Hg) and reducing the LVEDP (15 mm Hg); this stabilizes the patient sufficiently for definitive treatment.

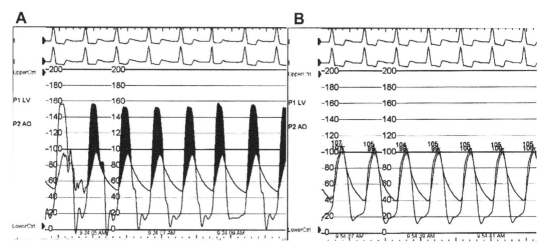

Fig. 6. Increase in pulse pressure post-TAVI with the presence of moderate postprocedural AR. (*A*) Pre-TAVI: severe pure AS; mean gradient = 48 mm Hg; AVA = 0.6 cm²; pulse pressure = 40 mm Hg. (*B*) Post-TAVI: relief of AS, moderate AR; mean gradient = 6 mm Hg; AVA = 1.8 cm²; pulse pressure = 60 mm Hg. Diastolic pressure dropped from 50 mm Hg to 40 mm Hg.

increase in aortic pulse pressure can signify important AR, but wide pulse pressure is generally a feature of chronic AR. Diastasis, the equalization of end-diastolic LV pressure and aortic diastolic pressure, is more indicative of acute severe AR (see **Fig. 7**).

The presence of severe AR post TAVI prompts an urgent evaluation of the etiology by echocardiography to guide therapy. If transvalvular, a second "bail-out" valve-in-valve should be considered.[26] If paravalvular, one may consider valve-in-valve or postdilatation with rapid pacing. If paravalvular in the setting of a low Medtronic CoreValve implant, one may consider snaring and upward traction of the prosthesis to bring the proximal covered skirt back and seal the annulus.[27]

POSTIMPLANT GRADIENT, VALVE AREA, AND PROSTHESIS-PATIENT MISMATCH

Incomplete stent-frame expansion is not uncommon following TAVI, particularly in the setting of heavy calcification.[28] Aggressive postdilatation is not a benign procedural step, and can potentially cause leaflet injury and device embolization. Moreover, good bioprosthetic hemodynamic function and a favorable clinical course may be seen despite incomplete stent expansion.[28] This scenario is particularly relevant for the long stent frame of the self-expanding design, as only a short 8- to 10-mm segment of the frame carries the valve; for this reason, postdilatation should be reserved for cases where hemodynamic function

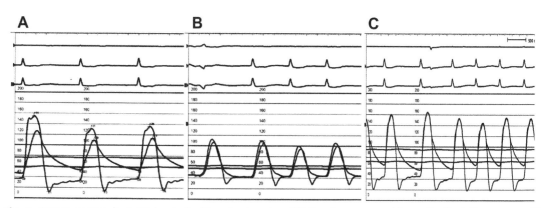

Fig. 7. Severe postimplant AR treated with valve-in-valve. (*A*) Baseline: severe AS; aortic diastolic pressure 40 mm Hg; LVEDP 20 mm Hg. (*B*) Post-TAVI #1: aortic diastolic pressure 20 mm Hg; LVEDP 20 mm Hg (ie, diastasis); severe paravalvular AR. (*C*) Valve-in-valve implantation: aortic diastolic pressure 40 mm Hg; LVEDP 20 mm Hg. Complete resolution of aortic valve gradient and AR.

Box 1
Causes of post-TAVI hypotension

Vascular complications—iliac rupture

Acute valve dysfunction

Coronary artery obstruction

Multiple rapid pacing episodes in patients with patients with poor LV function

is suboptimal on echocardiographic or transcatheter assessment.

Doppler echocardiography is known to correlate well with transcatheter measures of bioprosthetic gradients.[29] However, the Doppler peak instantaneous gradient is greater than the invasively determined peak-to-peak gradient, and use of mean gradients is preferable for evaluation.[30] Valve gradients can vary with changing loading conditions, and valve areas calculated by continuity equation or Gorlin equation are preferred for hemodynamic evaluation post implant. In the presence of a nondilated aorta, the phenomenon of pressure recovery in the proximal ascending aorta can mean that effective orifice area

calculated by continuity equation may be underestimated relative to that obtained by the Gorlin equation,[30] and hence a baseline immediate post-procedural transcatheter calculation is extremely useful for subsequent comparison.

For conventional surgical bioprostheses, prosthesis-patient mismatch (P-PM) is an important hemodynamic phenomenon, predicting diminished exercise tolerance, early bioprosthetic failure, and mortality. There are data showing lower incidences of P-PM with both principal TAVI designs relative to conventional bioprostheses,[3–5] and some evidence that optimal device positioning may reduce the incidence of P-PM.[4] The prognostic importance of post-TAVI P-PM remains unclear.

ASSESSMENT OF HYPOTENSION FOLLOWING TAVI

Post-TAVI AR has been discussed and is an important cause of postimplant hypotension (**Box 1**). Following Edwards TAVI and rapid pacing, either ventricular arrhythmia or myocardial stunning may occur and cause hemodynamic compromise (**Fig. 8**). Coronary ischemia may also cause

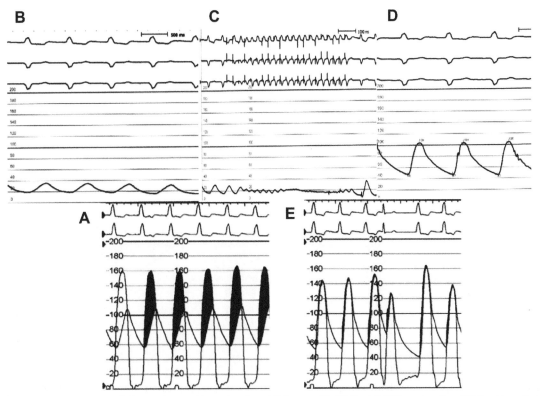

Fig. 8. Post-BAV myocardial stunning and hypotension. (*A*) Severe AS. (*B*) Post-BAV hypotension. (*C*) Rapid pacing for TAVI deployment. (*D*) Rapid recovery of normotension 1 minute later. (*E*) Final waveform with complete resolution of gradient.

myocardial depression (**Fig. 9**), and this may occur through displacement of native valvular calcium, causing left mainstem occlusion; the authors have employed prophylactic left mainstem cannulation and guidewire access to protect against this eventuality in the setting of a bulky, heavily calcified native aortic valve.

Particularly in the setting of postimplant hypotension, failure of the bioprosthetic leaflets to close may rarely result,[31] and can be resolved either by pushing the leaflets with a retrograde pigtail, by a period of cardiopulmonary bypass support, or by valve-in-valve; this has been seen with the Edwards Sapien design, as the default leaflet position is open, and has prompted a change in leaflet design in the Sapien XT to a default partially closed configuration. The Medtronic CoreValve leaflets are closed by default, which may make it favorable for the hemodynamically unstable or hypotensive patient.

Native leaflet overhang can occur after Edwards Sapien implantation, and can cause supravalvular obstruction. Acute severe mitral insufficiency may arise from the superstiff wire becoming entangled in the mitral subvalvular apparatus or, through deep implantation, encroachment onto the

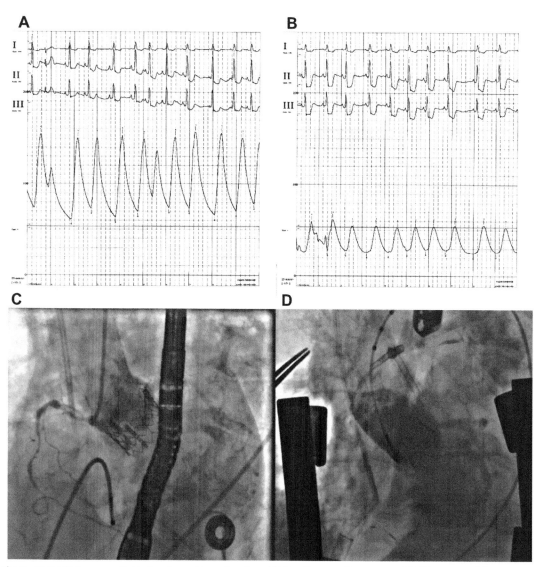

Fig. 9. Post-TAVI myocardial ischemia and hypotension. (*A*) Baseline, aortic pressure 152/69 mm Hg. (*B*) Post-TAVI, aortic pressure 55/26 mm Hg with ischemic electrocardiogram noted. (*C*) Angiography revealed left mainstem compromise with semi-occlusive displacement of calcified nodule from aortic valve. (*D*) Problem resolved with cardiopulmonary bypass, device explantation, and open aortic valve replacement.

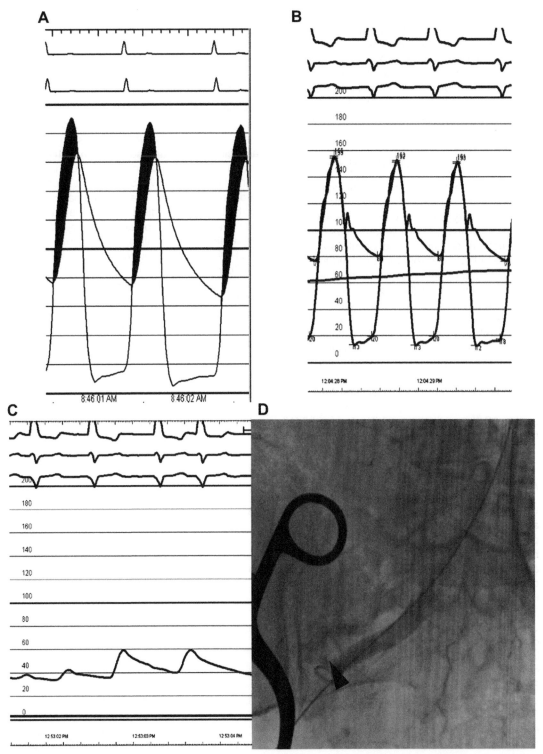

Fig. 10. Post-TAVI decreased cardiac output despite optimal valve hemodynamics: vascular complication. (*A*) Pre-TAVI: severe AS; cardiac output by thermodilution 3.1 L/min/m^2; mean AV gradient 34 mm Hg; AVA 0.75 cm^2. (*B*) Excellent post-TAVI hemodynamics, with resolution of AV gradient. Despite this, cardiac output was 1.2 L/min/m^2, an early demonstration of ensuing hemodynamic compromise. (*C*) On sheath removal, systolic blood pressure dropped to 50 mm Hg. (*D*) Peripheral arteriogram demonstrates an iliac perforation (*arrowhead* points to site of leak).

anterior mitral valve leaflet; this may be noted rapidly either on echocardiography or, if a Swan-Ganz catheter is in situ, with the development of CV waves on the pulmonary wedge. A postimplant low cardiac output assessment despite favorable transaortic hemodynamics can point to extracardiac causes, such as peripheral vascular complications (**Fig. 10**) or gastrointestinal bleeding.

HEMODYNAMIC SUPPORT DURING TAVI

Although counter to the ethos of a minimally invasive, catheter laboratory based intervention, cardiopulmonary support can be life-saving in the setting of the rare but serious hemodynamic complications described, and should always be available in the same room as the TAVI intervention, with additional venous access ready in situ.[32,33] TandemHeart (Cardiac Assist Inc, Pittsburgh, PA, USA), a percutaneous LV assist device, has been used in the setting of TAVI with the Medtronic CoreValve device[34,35] but, as it necessitates large-bore transseptal access, has been associated with hemodynamically important iatrogenic atrial septal defect.[36] The Impella 2.5 percutaneous device (Abiomed Inc, Danvers, MA, USA) has been used successfully even in the setting of severe AS,[37] and is a possibility for post-TAVI hemodynamic support in the event of instability.

ANESTHESIA AND TAVI HEMODYNAMICS

Use of anesthesia in TAVI is a subject for debate as, although it causes myocardial depression, potentially contributing to hemodynamic instability, it protects the airway with optimal positive airways ventilation should pulmonary edema occur. Rapid extubation in the cardiac catheter laboratory or shortly after is a priority, particularly in the elderly patient. Other issues governing the decision for general anesthesia are the method of access and whether transesophageal imaging is required. For transfemoral TAVI, use of percutaneous preclosure devices such as Prostar or Perclose (Abbott Vascular, Redwood City, CA, USA) is now the standard of care for the Medtronic CoreValve device, allowing the possibility of a procedure under local anesthesia with light sedation[35,38] and only fluoroscopy required for imaging given the 53- to 55-mm stent frame; such preclosing techniques are increasingly used for the Edwards Sapien valve.[39] The requirement for TEE with this device, given its 14- to 16-mm stent frame, with a consequent greater need for precise implantation, is another factor influencing the use of anesthesia; nevertheless, some centers have reported TEE with light sedation for the TAVI procedure.[40]

SUMMARY

The hemodynamics of TAVI appear to be at least as good as conventional aortic bioprostheses. Hemodynamic maneuvers, such as intraprocedural pacing at rates around 100 bpm, can be helpful in reducing the clinical impact of acute intraprocedural AR, particularly if bradycardia is present, by shortening diastole. There is dramatic reduction of the LV-aortic gradient both by the transfemoral and transapical approach and by both self-expanding and balloon-expandable designs. Post-TAVI diastolic, pulse pressure, and LV end-diastolic pressure may increase, decrease, or remain unchanged depending on pre-TAVI and post-TAVI AR, and the prompt appreciation of such trends can be useful early clues to a malfunctioning valve or a developing complication intraprocedurally.

REFERENCES

1. De Paulis R, Schmitz C, Scaffa R, et al. In vitro evaluation of aortic valve prosthesis in a novel valved conduit with pseudosinuses of Valsalva. J Thorac Cardiovasc Surg 2005;130:1016–21.
2. Ruel J, Lachance G. A new bioreactor for the development of tissue-engineered heart valves. Ann Biomed Eng 2009;37:674–81.
3. Clavel MA, Webb JG, Pibarot P, et al. Comparison of the hemodynamic performance of percutaneous and surgical bioprostheses for the treatment of severe aortic stenosis. J Am Coll Cardiol 2009;53:1883–91.
4. Jilaihawi H, Chin D, Spyt T, et al. Prosthesis-patient mismatch after transcatheter aortic valve implantation with the Medtronic-Corevalve bioprosthesis. Eur Heart J 2010;31:857–64.
5. Tzikas A, Piazza N, Geleijnse ML, et al. Prosthesis-patient mismatch after transcatheter aortic valve implantation with the Medtronic CoreValve system in patients with aortic stenosis. Am J Cardiol 2010; 106:255–60.
6. Grube E, Buellesfeld L, Mueller R, et al. Progress and current status of percutaneous aortic valve replacement: results of three device generations of the CoreValve Revalving system. Circ Cardiovasc Interv 2008;1:167–75.
7. Walther T, Schuler G, Borger MA, et al. Transapical aortic valve implantation in 100 consecutive patients: comparison to propensity-matched conventional aortic valve replacement. Eur Heart J 2010;31: 1398–403.

8. Hatle L, Angelsen BA, Tromsdal A. Non-invasive assessment of aortic stenosis by Doppler ultrasound. Br Heart J 1980;43:284–92.

9. Hegrenaes L, Hatle L. Aortic stenosis in adults. Noninvasive estimation of pressure differences by continuous wave Doppler echocardiography. Br Heart J 1985;54:396–404.

10. Currie PJ, Seward JB, Reeder GS, et al. Continuous-wave Doppler echocardiographic assessment of severity of calcific aortic stenosis: a simultaneous Doppler-catheter correlative study in 100 adult patients. Circulation 1985;71:1162–9.

11. Bonow RO, Carabello BA, Chatterjee K, et al. 2008 focused update incorporated into the ACC/AHA 2006 guidelines for the management of patients with valvular heart disease: a report of the American College of Cardiology/American Heart Association Task Force on Practice Guidelines (Writing Committee to revise the 1998 guidelines for the management of patients with valvular heart disease). Endorsed by the Society of Cardiovascular Anesthesiologists, Society for Cardiovascular Angiography and Interventions, and Society of Thoracic Surgeons. J Am Coll Cardiol 2008;52:e1–142.

12. Turi ZG. Whom do you trust? Misguided faith in the catheter- or Doppler-derived aortic valve gradient. Catheter Cardiovasc Interv 2005;65:180–2.

13. Carabello BA, Barry WH, Grossman W. Changes in arterial pressure during left heart pullback in patients with aortic stenosis: a sign of severe aortic stenosis. Am J Cardiol 1979;44:424–7.

14. Stoebe T, Adicoff A, Weir EK, et al. Simultaneous measurement of aortic and left ventricular pressures in aortic stenosis using a double lumen pigtail catheter. Cathet Cardiovasc Diagn 1984;10:515–7.

15. Bae JH, Lerman A, Yang E, et al. Feasibility of a pressure wire and single arterial puncture for assessing aortic valve area in patients with aortic stenosis. J Invasive Cardiol 2006;18:359–62.

16. Gordon JB, Folland ED. Analysis of aortic valve gradients by transseptal technique: implications for noninvasive evaluation. Cathet Cardiovasc Diagn 1989;17:144–51.

17. Suh WM, Witzke CF, Palacios IF. Suicide left ventricle following transcatheter aortic valve implantation. Catheter Cardiovasc Interv 2010;76(4):616–20.

18. Kayalar N, Schaff HV, Daly RC, et al. Concomitant septal myectomy at the time of aortic valve replacement for severe aortic stenosis. Ann Thorac Surg 2010;89:459–64.

19. Moreno R, Calvo L, Garcia E, et al. Severe septal hypertrophy: is it necessarily a contraindication for the transcatheter implantation of an Edwards-Sapien prosthesis? Rev Esp Cardiol 2010;63:241–2.

20. Jilaihawi H, Jeilan M, Spyt T, et al. Early regression of left ventricular wall thickness following percutaneous aortic valve replacement with the CoreValve bioprosthesis. J Invasive Cardiol 2009;21:151–5 [discussion: 156–8].

21. Finkelstein A, Keren G, Banai S. Treatment of severe valvular aortic stenosis and subvalvular discrete subaortic stenosis and septal hypertrophy with percutaneous CoreValve aortic valve implantation. Catheter Cardiovasc Interv 2010;75:801–3.

22. Webb JG, Pasupati S, Achtem L, et al. Rapid pacing to facilitate transcatheter prosthetic heart valve implantation. Catheter Cardiovasc Interv 2006;68:199–204.

23. Kapadia SR, Goel SS, Yuksel U, et al. Lessons learned from balloon aortic valvuloplasty experience from the pre-transcatheter aortic valve implantation era. J Interv Cardiol 2010;23(5):499–508.

24. Moussa ID. Balloon aortic valvuloplasty: time for re-evaluation of when and how. Catheter Cardiovasc Interv 2010;75:799–800.

25. Shen WF, Roubin GS, Hirasawa K, et al. Noninvasive assessment of acute effects of nifedipine on rest and exercise hemodynamics and cardiac function in patients with aortic regurgitation. J Am Coll Cardiol 1984;4:902–7.

26. Rodes-Cabau J, Dumont E, Doyle D. "Valve-in-valve" for the treatment of paravalvular leaks following transcatheter aortic valve implantation. Catheter Cardiovasc Interv 2009;74:1116–9.

27. Vavouranakis M, Vrachatis DA, Toutouzas KP, et al. "Bail out" procedures for malpositioning of aortic valve prosthesis (CoreValve). Int J Cardiol 2010;145(1):154–5.

28. Schultz CJ, Weustink A, Piazza N, et al. Geometry and degree of apposition of the CoreValve ReValving system with multislice computed tomography after implantation in patients with aortic stenosis. J Am Coll Cardiol 2009;54:911–8.

29. Burstow DJ, Nishimura RA, Bailey KR, et al. Continuous wave Doppler echocardiographic measurement of prosthetic valve gradients. A simultaneous Doppler-catheter correlative study. Circulation 1989;80:504–14.

30. Bach DS. Echo/Doppler evaluation of hemodynamics after aortic valve replacement: principles of interrogation and evaluation of high gradients. JACC Cardiovasc Imaging 2010;3:296–304.

31. Pasupati S, Puri A, Devlin G, et al. Transcatheter aortic valve implantation complicated by acute structural valve failure requiring immediate valve in valve implantation. Heart Lung Circ 2010;19(10):611–4.

32. Al-Attar N, Ghodbane W, Himbert D, et al. Unexpected complications of transapical aortic valve implantation. Ann Thorac Surg 2009;88:90–4.

33. Masson JB, Kovac J, Schuler G, et al. Transcatheter aortic valve implantation: review of the nature, management, and avoidance of procedural complications. JACC Cardiovasc Interv 2009;2:811–20.

34. Piazza N, Serruys PW, de Jaegere P. Feasibility of complex coronary intervention in combination with percutaneous aortic valve implantation in patients with aortic stenosis using percutaneous left ventricular assist device (TandemHeart). Catheter Cardiovasc Interv 2009;73:161–6.

35. Grube E, Schuler G, Buellesfeld L, et al. Percutaneous aortic valve replacement for severe aortic stenosis in high-risk patients using the second- and current third-generation self-expanding CoreValve prosthesis: device success and 30-day clinical outcome. J Am Coll Cardiol 2007;50:69–76.

36. Sur JP, Pagani FD, Moscucci M. Percutaneous closure of an iatrogenic atrial septal defect. Catheter Cardiovasc Interv 2009;73:267–71.

37. Harjai KJ, O'Neill WW. Hemodynamic support using the Impella 2.5 catheter system during high-risk percutaneous coronary intervention in a patient with severe aortic stenosis. J Interv Cardiol 2010;23:66–9.

38. Behan M, Haworth P, Hutchinson N, et al. Percutaneous aortic valve implants under sedation: our initial experience. Catheter Cardiovasc Interv 2008;72:1012–5.

39. Kahlert P, Eggebrecht H, Erbel R, et al. A modified "preclosure" technique after percutaneous aortic valve replacement. Catheter Cardiovasc Interv 2008;72:877–84.

40. Ben-Dor I, Waksman R, Satler L, et al. Edwards-Sapien aortic valve: transfemoral approach. Vascular Disease Management 2010;7:E1–9.

The Pulmonary Valve

Kevin P. Fitzgerald, MD[a,b], Michael J. Lim, MD, FSCAI[b,*]

KEYWORDS

- Pulmonary stenosis • Valvuloplasty • Echocardiogram
- Catheterization

The pulmonary valve consists of 3 leaflets and is similar in anatomy to the aortic valve. It is the least likely to be affected by acquired disease, and thus, most disorders are congenital. The most common hemodynamic abnormality is the congenitally narrowed domed valve of pulmonic stenosis. A minority of individuals may have a thickened or dysplastic valve. Infundibular hypertrophy may present as pulmonic stenosis with normal valve structures. Occasionally, ventricular septal defects also accompany the deformed valve. Pulmonary valvular (and subvalvular and supravalvular) lesions are diagnosed by echocardiography, pressure recordings of the right side of the heart, and right ventricular angiography.[1–6] Although uncommon, it is important to recognize the different waveforms associated with pulmonary stenosis, pulmonary regurgitation, and conditions that may mimic or be confused for pulmonary stenosis in the absence of true valvular abnormalities.

PULMONARY STENOSIS

Obstruction of right ventricular outflow can occur at 3 locations in relation to the pulmonary valve: subvalvular, supravalvular, and valvular. Obstructions at all the 3 locations are represented by a step-up in pressure between the right ventricle and the main pulmonary artery. Subvalvular stenosis is also known as infundibular pulmonary stenosis and is secondary to fibromuscular narrowing or right ventricular hypertrophy. Supravalvular stenosis is also known as pulmonary artery stenosis or peripheral pulmonary stenosis and is caused by narrowing of the pulmonary artery or its branches. This condition can be associated with Williams syndrome. Stenosis of the pulmonary valve is virtually always congenital and can be associated with Noonan syndrome, congenital rubella, or tetralogy of Fallot. Acquired pulmonary valve stenosis can be secondary to carcinoid syndrome or, rarely, rheumatic fever.

Clinical Evaluation

Mild pulmonary valve stenosis is well tolerated with little clinical sequela. Patients with moderate pulmonary stenosis may begin to have symptoms of dyspnea on exertion. As the pulmonary stenosis progresses to the severe form, the right ventricular wall stress increases leading to right ventricle hypertrophy. Severe pulmonary stenosis eventually leads to right ventricular failure, and these patients complain of dyspnea, lower extremity swelling, and abdominal fullness. The limited right ventricular stroke volume seen in severe pulmonary stenosis can lead to exertional symptoms of dyspnea, angina, and syncope. The physical examination in severe pulmonary stenosis shows a prominent jugular venous a wave as the atrium contracts against a thickened and noncompliant right ventricle. There may also be liver congestion, edema, and ascites. A right ventricular heave may be appreciated on palpation of the chest wall. The murmur of pulmonary stenosis is a crescendo and decrescendo systolic ejection murmur heard best over the left upper sternal border. As the pulmonary stenosis increases in severity, the peak of the murmur occurs later in the systole, and the pulmonary component of the second heart sound gets softer. The second heart sound is widely split, but eventually, the A_2 of the second heart sound may become difficult to appreciate because the murmur peaks late and obscures the A_2.

a Comprehensive Cardiology Consultants, Crestview Hills, KY, USA
b Division of Cardiology, Department of Internal Medicine, Saint Louis University School of Medicine, 3635 Vista Avenue, 13th Floor, Desloge Towers, St Louis, MO 63110-0250, USA
* Corresponding author.
E-mail address: limmj@slu.edu

Cardiol Clin 29 (2011) 223–227
doi:10.1016/j.ccl.2011.01.006

Echocardiography

On 2-dimensional echocardiography, patients with pulmonary stenosis may show evidence of right ventricular hypertrophy, right ventricular enlargement, or right atrial enlargement. Right ventricular pressure overload produces flattening of the interventricular septum during systole and diastole. The pulmonary valve leaflets are typically domed and thickened and demonstrate fused leaflets with incompletely formed raphae. Subvalvular stenosis can be present secondary to hypertrophy of the right ventricular infundibulum. Color flow Doppler imaging demonstrates high-velocity turbulent systolic flow through the pulmonary valve. There may also be coexisting tricuspid regurgitation because of elevated right ventricular systolic pressure. On continuous wave Doppler, the pulmonary stenosis is severe when the maximum pulmonary valve velocity exceeds 4 m/s during systole (transvalvular pressure gradient of 64 mm Hg using the modified Bernoulli equation).

Cardiac Catheterization

If the patient is a candidate for pulmonary valvuloplasty and the pulmonary valve peak Doppler velocity on the echocardiogram is greater than 3 m/s, cardiac catheterization is warranted. During catheterization of the right side of the heart and angiography, special attention should be paid to the subvalvular and supravalvular regions. The exact location of the pressure gradient should be sought to distinguish valvular from extravalvular stenosis because a dynamic right ventricular outflow tract obstruction from a hypertrophied right ventricle could cause significant hypotension after successful balloon valvuloplasty. Angiography may demonstrate the systolic doming or cone shape of the restricted pulmonary valve leaflets. Heavy calcification of the pulmonary valve leaflets is rare, so radiographic imaging of the stenotic pulmonary valve is difficult.

Treatment

In patients requiring intervention for pulmonary stenosis, the treatment of choice is balloon valvuloplasty. The usual lack of calcified leaflets in pulmonary stenosis allows for effective splitting of the fused leaflets. Patients with dysplastic valves, such as in Noonan syndrome, or those with subvalvular stenosis are not ideal candidates for balloon valvuloplasty and should be considered for surgical valvuloplasty. Balloon valvuloplasty is usually performed with a long polyethylene balloon or an Inoue balloon (Toray International America Inc, Houston, TX, USA). A successful balloon valvuloplasty usually completely eliminates the pulmonary valve pressure gradient. If patients become hypotensive secondary to an unrecognized dynamic right ventricular outflow obstruction from right ventricular hypertrophy, they should receive aggressive intravenous fluid administration and β-blocker therapy. Eventually, the right ventricular hypertrophy should regress after the pressure gradient across the pulmonary valve has been relieved. Follow-up data up to 10 years out suggest that balloon valvuloplasty has equivalent outcomes to surgical valvuloplasty. After surgical or balloon valvuloplasty, mild and clinically insignificant pulmonary regurgitation is common.

PULMONARY REGURGITATION

Trace or physiologic pulmonary valve regurgitation can often be found in a normal heart without a pathologic condition or pulmonary hypertension. Pathologic pulmonary valve regurgitation is usually caused by dilation of either the pulmonary valve annulus or the pulmonary artery, secondary to pulmonary hypertension, idiopathic pulmonary artery dilation, or connective tissue disease. Rarely, congenital absence of a pulmonary valve leaflet may cause regurgitation. Iatrogenic causes include pulmonary valve trauma related to balloon valvuloplasty, pulmonary artery catheters, or surgical repair of congenital heart disease.

Clinical Evaluation

In the absence of pulmonary hypertension, pulmonary regurgitation may be well tolerated for many years. Severe pulmonary regurgitation leads to signs and symptoms of right ventricular overload. If the pulmonary regurgitation is secondary to underlying pulmonary hypertension, various symptoms may be present depending on the pulmonary artery pressures. Initially, the patient may only complain of exertional dyspnea or fatigue. Dyspnea at rest, edema, ascites, angina, and even syncope may occur as the pulmonary hypertension progresses in severity.

Right ventricular volume and pressure overload may lead to right ventricular heave, a right-sided third or fourth heart sound, elevated jugular venous pressure, liver congestion, ascites, and edema. There may also be a widened split of the second heart sound because of an increase in the right ventricular stroke volume.

The murmur of pulmonary regurgitation is usually a diastolic decrescendo blowing murmur auscultated best at the left upper sternal border. When pulmonary hypertension is absent, the murmur is low to medium pitched. If the systolic pulmonary artery pressure is greater than 55 mm Hg, the

Graham Steell murmur may be present, which includes a prominent P$_2$ of the second heart sound followed by a diastolic, high-pitched, blowing murmur caused by the large diastolic pressure gradient between the pulmonary artery and the right ventricle.

Echocardiography

The echocardiographic diagnosis of pulmonary regurgitation is usually made via color flow Doppler imaging using a transthoracic parasternal short axis view at the base of the heart. Pulmonary regurgitation appears as a diastolic jet traveling retrograde through the pulmonary valve and into the right ventricular outflow tract. The color jet of severe pulmonary regurgitation usually fills the right ventricular outflow tract.

Continuous wave spectral Doppler in the parasternal short axis view can also be used. Pulmonary regurgitation appears as a diastolic down-sloping velocity curve traveling toward the ultrasound transducer. Severe pulmonary regurgitation has a dense Doppler velocity signal representing a high density of regurgitant red blood cells. The slope of the regurgitant flow signal also represents the severity and acuity of the pulmonary regurgitation. Steeper slopes represent more-severe and/or more-acute-onset regurgitation, implying elevated right ventricular end-diastolic pressures. Using the modified Bernoulli equation, the pulmonary artery diastolic pressure can be calculated using the velocity of the pulmonary artery regurgitation jet at end diastole as

$$PADP = 4 \times (\text{velocity of PR at end diastole})^2 + \text{right atrial pressure}$$

where PADP is the pulmonary artery diastolic pressure and PR denotes the pulmonary artery.

Indirect echocardiographic evidence of pulmonary valve regurgitation severity includes right ventricular enlargement (> two-thirds of the left ventricular size) and right ventricular volume overload (diastolic flattening of the interventricular septum).

Cardiac Catheterization

Angiographic imaging of pulmonary regurgitation involves crossing the pulmonary valve with a balloon-tipped or pigtail pulmonary catheter and then injecting contrast into the proximal pulmonary artery. The pulmonary catheter interrupts normal coaptation of the pulmonary leaflets and can thus cause artifactual pulmonary regurgitation. Because of the superiority of echocardiography, angiographic evaluation of pulmonary regurgitation is rarely performed. In the setting of

severe pulmonary regurgitation, hemodynamic measurements may reveal pulmonary artery hypertension, a widened pulmonary artery pulse pressure, and an elevated end-diastolic pressure with a steep upward slope.

CASE PRESENTATIONS
Case 1

A 60-year-old woman presented with acute onset of right-sided hemiparesis and was treated with tissue plasminogen activator for an acute middle cerebral artery ischemic stroke. In a workup for a potential cardiac source of emboli, she was found to have an atrial septal defect (ASD) and elevated right ventricular pressure by echocardiography (estimated right ventricular systolic pressure of 96 mm Hg). She was sent to the catheterization laboratory for evaluation of pulmonary hypertension, and catheterization of the right side of the heart was performed. **Fig. 1** shows a pullback from the pulmonary artery into the right ventricle. The systolic pulmonary pressure was observed to be about 25 mm Hg, and the pressure tracing then jumped to a right ventricular pressure of about 115 mm Hg. This pullback was observed under fluoroscopy to note where the change in pressure occurred, and it was found that the catheter crossed the pulmonic valve at the same time when the premature contractions were seen, and a subsequent increase in systolic pressure was seen. Right ventriculography was performed (**Fig. 2**), showing signs of pulmonic leaflet doming (consistent with valvular stenosis) and resultant infundibular hypertrophy and narrowing. **Fig. 3** shows the right ventricular pressure. Close inspection shows a steep increase in the diastolic portion of the waveform, consistent with altered right ventricular compliance. This steep increase in the diastolic portion of the ventricular waveform has been implicated in the resultant increase in right atrial pressure, resulting in an increased risk for

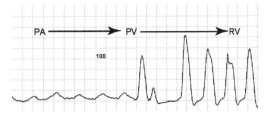

Fig. 1. Pullback from the pulmonary artery (PA) to the right ventricle (RV) through a 7F Swan-Ganz catheter on a 100-mm Hg scale showing a 70-mm Hg gradient in a patient with valvular pulmonary stenosis. PV, pulmonary vein.

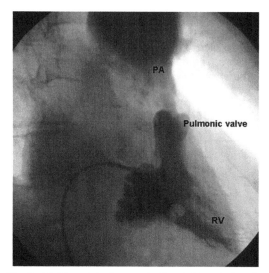

Fig. 2. Right ventriculogram in the right anterior oblique projection through a Berman catheter, demonstrating pulmonic valve narrowing and doming of the leaflets, infundibular hypertrophy, and tricuspid regurgitation. PA, pulmonary artery; RV, right ventricle.

paradoxic emboli across an ASD or patent foramen ovale.

Although data obtained in this case were effective in establishing the diagnosis of a clear gradient across the pulmonic valve and outflow tract, they were obtained with a single catheter only. Most operators prefer to measure simultaneous pressures with 2 separate catheters under careful fluoroscopic guidance to pinpoint the exact location of the gradient. This approach is especially important

when considering balloon valvuloplasty because patients with a predominant infundibular gradient ultimately respond poorly.

Case 2

A 26-year old man presented with a syncopal episode. On clinical evaluation, he was found to have a significant systolic murmur. Echocardiography was then performed showing that he had a bicuspid aortic valve without significant gradient. In addition, there was significant pulmonary hypertension (with an estimated right ventricular systolic pressure of 100 mm Hg) and a gradient of 64 mm Hg across the pulmonic valve. Close inspection of the pulmonic valve and outflow tract showed some subvalvular hypertrophy, but the valve leaflets themselves were thickened and showed the classic doming appearance, consistent with valvular pulmonic stenosis.

Given this finding of symptomatic severe pulmonary stenosis, he was taken to the catheterization laboratory for confirmation of the diagnosis and pulmonary valvuloplasty. Pressures were measured and found to be as follows: mean right atrial pressure, 4 mm Hg; mean pulmonary capillary wedge pressure, 12 mm Hg; and aortic pressure, 100/70 mm Hg. His Fick cardiac output was calculated to be 6.1 L/min. His baseline gradient was obtained with an 8F dual-lumen pigtail catheter across the pulmonic valve (**Fig. 4**). The current classification of pulmonary stenosis considers a gradient less than 30 mm Hg to be mild, a gradient of 30 to 50 mm Hg to be moderate, and a gradient (such as in this case) greater than 50 mm Hg to be severe.[7]

Pulmonic valvuloplasty is now the preferred treatment for patients such as the one described. In fact, invasively obtained peak-to-peak gradients greater than 60 mm Hg in asymptomatic patients or greater than 50 mm Hg in symptomatic patients constitute the Class I recommendations for treatment with

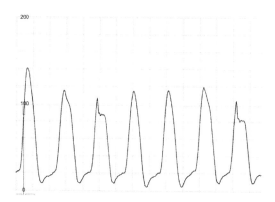

Fig. 3. Right ventricular pressure tracing on a 200-mm Hg scale, demonstrating a marked increase in normal right ventricular systolic pressure in a patient with pulmonic stenosis. Focusing on the diastolic portion of the pressure tracing reveals a steep increase in the right ventricular diastolic pressure, consistent with altered right ventricular compliance.

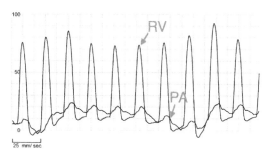

Fig. 4. Simultaneously obtained pulmonary artery (PA) and right ventricular (RV) pressures demonstrating a large peak-to-peak gradient across the pulmonic valve, consistent with severe pulmonic stenosis.

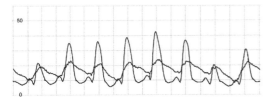

Fig. 5. Simultaneously obtained pulmonary artery and right ventricular pressures after successful pulmonary balloon valvuloplasty on a 50-mm Hg scale. The right ventricular systolic pressure has decreased from 80 to 35 mm Hg, and the pulmonary arterial pressure remains at about 20 mm Hg, leaving a residual 15-mm Hg gradient.

balloon valvuloplasty.[7] These recommendations are principally based on the observations that significant long-lasting reductions in the pulmonic gradient could be achieved with low morbidity and mortality. Specifically, Chen and colleagues[8] showed that in 53 patients, pulmonary balloon valvuloplasty decreased right ventricular pressures from 91 ± 46 mm Hg to 38 ± 32 mm Hg acutely. After a mean period of 7 ± 3 years of follow-up, the gradient across the valve remained low, with only 13% of patients having postprocedural pulmonary insufficiency.

The patient underwent pulmonary valvuloplasty with sequential dilation of the valve, and the hemodynamic tracing (**Fig. 5**) was obtained. At this point, given the marked reduction of the gradient, the procedure was stopped. This case, as in most, demonstrates that there is a residual pulmonic gradient. A persistent systolic gradient suggests that subvalvular stenosis of the right ventricular outflow tract may be present. The reduction in systolic gradient at follow-up examination of the patients undergoing pulmonary valvuloplasty suggests that a delayed reduction of the gradient produces results similar to those of surgical pulmonic valvulotomy and that the systolic gradient measured immediately after balloon valvuloplasty underestimates the long-term results of the procedure. This finding also supports the idea that stenosis of the infundibulum is not an absolute contraindication to percutaneous balloon pulmonic valvuloplasty.

Although the mechanism of infundibular tract systolic gradients is incompletely understood, subvalvular muscular hypertrophy and activity of contraction in the unrestrained phase immediately on relief of valvular resistance probably produce a hyperkinetic effect. Therapy with β-blockers has been recommended, although in most adult series these medications were not necessary.

SUMMARY

Pulmonary stenosis is predominantly a congenital disorder and is also usually well tolerated in its mild and moderate forms. Invasive hemodynamics is principally performed in conjunction with pulmonic valvuloplasty for patients with significant gradients, with or without symptoms. Patients requiring pulmonic balloon valvuloplasty have high rates of procedural success and long-term clinical success.

REFERENCES

1. Grossman W. Profiles in valvular heart disease. In: Grossman W, editor. Cardiac catheterization and angiography. Boston: Lea & Febiger; 1986. p. 359–81.
2. Freed MD, Keane JR. Profiles in congenital heart disease. In: Grossman W, editor. Cardiac catheterization and angiography. Boston: Lea & Febiger; 1986. p. 446–69.
3. Hirshfeld JW. Valve function: stenosis and insufficiency. In: Pepine CJ, editor. Diagnostic and therapeutic cardiac catheterization. Baltimore (MD): Williams & Wilkins; 1989. p. 390–410.
4. Conti CR. Cardiac catheterization and the patient with congenital heart disease. In: Pepine CJ, editor. Diagnostic and therapeutic cardiac catheterization. Baltimore (MD): Williams & Wilkins; 1989. p. 508–22.
5. Hayes CJ, Gersony WM, Driscoll DJ. Second natural history study of congenital heart defects. Results of treatment of patients with pulmonary valvular stenosis. Circulation 1993;87(Suppl 2):128–37.
6. Bashore T. Adult congenital heart disease: right ventricular outflow tract lesions. Circulation 2007; 115(14):1933–47.
7. Warnes CA, Williams RG, Bashore TM, et al. ACC/AHA 2008 guidelines for the management of adults with congenital heart disease: a report of the American College of Cardiology/American Heart Association Task Force on Practice Guidelines (Writing Committee to Develop Guidelines for the Management of Adults With Congenital Heart Disease). J Am Coll Cardiol 2008;52:143–263.
8. Chen C, Cheng T, Huang T, et al. Percutaneous balloon valvuloplasty for pulmonic stenosis in adolescents and adults. N Engl J Med 1996;335:21–5.

Prosthetic Heart Valves

C. Ryan Longnecker, MD, Michael J. Lim, MD, FSCAI*

KEYWORDS
- Prosthetic • Heart • Valve • Implant

The first prosthetic valve was implanted by Hufnagel[1] in 1952 in a patient with aortic insufficiency (AI). Since then, prosthetic valves have evolved into various mechanical and bioprosthetic shapes and sizes. Despite the excitement surrounding the current development of prosthetic heart valves, surgically implanted valves remain the mainstay of current practice, and this article discusses the hemodynamic issues associated with the more commonly placed valves.

Mechanical valves are synthetic and based on a ball-and-cage, tilting disk, or bileaflet design, with the bileaflet type being the most commonly implanted valves in the modern era. Bioprosthetic valves are composed mainly of living material and can be formed from porcine or bovine tissue, homografts (valves from other humans), or autografts (valve moved from one position to another in the same heart). A list of some of the US Food and Drug Administration–approved devices is found in **Table 1**.

When patients are being selected for valve replacement surgery, several variables play a role in deciding which type of device they will receive. Age, comorbidities (ie, renal dysfunction), child-bearing potential, occupation, medication compliance, fall risk, and bleeding histories all help determine the appropriate device. Mechanical valves have the advantage of potentially lasting a lifetime (>30 years), but the disadvantage of requiring chronic anticoagulation. Bioprosthetic valves do not require anticoagulation, but limited durability is a major drawback, with the need for rereplacement often occurring at 10 to 15 years. For more specifics regarding guidance of specific valve replacement surgeries, readers should consult the American College of Cardiology/American Heart Association guidelines for the management of patients with valvular heart disease.[2]

PHYSIOLOGIC CONSIDERATIONS

Valve replacement, whether in the aortic or mitral positions, replaces a stenotic and/or regurgitant valve with an improved, but imperfect, physiologic state. There are often significant changes in the patient's cardiac performance that developed prior to the valve replacement surgery and are irreversible. All prosthetic valves leave the patient with some degree of stenosis. As the valves are endothelialized or develop significant pannus formation, this stenosis may become worse. Device manufacturers have established normal baseline gradients based on the device type, size, and placement location; these values should be reviewed before determining abnormal gradients/function of any prosthetic valve. **Table 2** lists common valves and expected Doppler-derived mean gradients with each type. In the table, 23 mm has been chosen as the aortic valve size and 27 mm (except for the Starr-Edwards, which is 28 mm) as the mitral valve size for comparison. This shows the mild degree of stenosis inherent in the smaller effective orifice areas of prosthetic valves. In general, ball-and-cage valves have the highest mean gradients, followed by single-tilting disc, stented bioprostheses, bileaflet tilting discs, homografts, and stentless bioprostheses, respectively.

In conjunction with an intrinsic gradient resisting forward flow, all mechanical valves and some bioprosthetic valves also have a degree of regurgitation built into the design. This regurgitation ensures proper opening and closing of the valve and helps to keep clots/debris from forming on

Division of Cardiology, Department of Internal Medicine, Saint Louis University School of Medicine, 3635 Vista Avenue, 13th Floor, Desloge Towers, St Louis, MO 63110-0250, USA
* Corresponding author.
E-mail address: limmj@slu.edu

Cardiol Clin 29 (2011) 229–236
doi:10.1016/j.ccl.2011.01.007

Table 1
Commonly used prosthetic valves

Mechanical	Examples	First Year Released
Ball and cage	Starr-Edwards	1965
Tilting disk	Medtronic Hall, Omniscience, Bjork-Shiley[a]	1977
Bileaflet	St Jude, CarboMedics	1977
Bioprosthetic		
Porcine aortic valve[b]	Hancock, Carpentier-Edwards	1970
Bovine pericardial[b]	Carpentier-Edwards	1982
Stentless porcine[b]	Toronto Stentless, Freestyle	1991
Homograft	Human Cadaveric Aortic	1962
Autologous	Pulmonary autograft (Ross procedure)	1967

[a] No longer available because of problems with strut fractures and associated mortality.
[b] Heterografts.

the valve. After initial implantation, there may also be a small amount of paravalvular leak with prosthetic valves; this should be followed closely, but often closes without surgical intervention. Significant worsening of prosthetic regurgitation can result in a worsening of symptoms, and evaluation of the reverse flow is warranted.

HEMODYNAMIC ASSESSMENT OF IMPLANTED VALVES

Despite these accepted hemodynamic limitations of prosthetic valves, most of them function effectively for a long time. Clinically, it becomes challenging when a prosthetic valve is suspected of dysfunction in a patient. The hemodynamic assessment of prosthetic valves is mainly done by transthoracic and transesophageal echocardiography in current practice. Transthoracic echocardiography often allows for adequate visualization of the ventricular side of the valves, but acoustic shadowing inhibits the ability to see the atrial or aortic sides of the valves. Transesophageal echocardiography is superior in giving detail about these areas and also providing enhanced resolution of the valve structures. Both of these modalities can be used for Doppler assessment of the valvular gradients and can be followed over time to determine whether there has been progression of disease in those with abnormal valves (**Fig. 1**). Excellent correlation of echo-based and catheter-based hemodynamic findings has been shown,[3] leaving invasive hemodynamic assessment of valves to only the most challenging of cases. In particular, invasive hemodynamic prosthetic valve assessment is currently reserved for when the noninvasive data do not fit the clinical situation.

Catheter-based hemodynamics of prosthetic valves require experience and skill from the operator, because no 2 cases are exactly alike. The assessment of the left ventricular pressure measured across an aortic valve prosthesis may

Table 2
Expected valvular gradients for prosthetic valves

Mechanical	Aortic Position (Mean Gradient in mm Hg)	Mitral Position (Mean Gradient in mm Hg)
Starr-Edwards	21.98 ± 8.8	7 ± 2.75
Medtronic Hall	13.5 ± 4.79	NA
St Jude	13.77 ± 5.33	5 ± 1.82
Bioprosthetic		
Hancock	12.36 ± 3.82	5 ± 2
Carpentier-Edwards	13.01 ± 5.27	3.6
Toronto Stentless	7.08 ± 4.33	NA

Data from Rosenhek R, Binder T, Maurer G, et al. Normal values for Doppler echocardiographic assessment of heart valve prostheses. J Am Soc Echo 2003;16:1116–27.

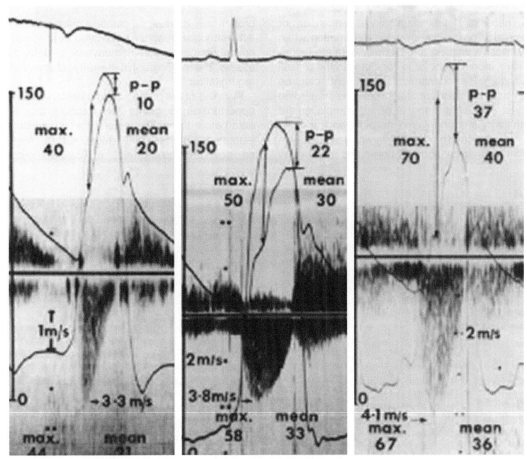

Fig. 1. Simultaneous Doppler pressure gradients and invasive hemodynamic waveforms showing equivalent data between both techniques for multiple prosthetic valves. (*From* Burstow DJ, Nishimura RA, Bailey KR, et al. Continuous wave Doppler echocardiographic measurements of prosthetic valve gradients. A simultaneous Doppler-catheter correlative study. Circulation 1989;80:510; with permission.)

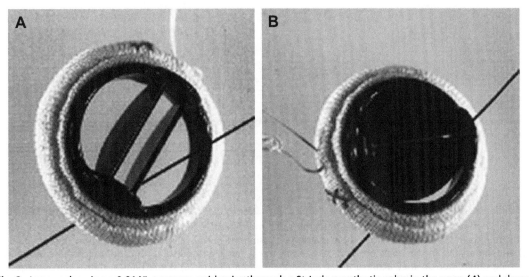

Fig. 2. Images showing a 0.014″ pressure guidewire through a St Jude prosthetic valve in the open (*A*) and closed (*B*) position. Please see text for specific details. (*From* Parham W, El Shafei A, Rajjoub H, et al. Retrograde left ventricular hemodynamic assessment across bileaflet prosthetic aortic valves: the use of a high-fidelity pressure sensor angioplasty guidewire. Catheter Cardiovasc Interv 2003;59:512; with permission.)

be necessary for diagnosing pericardial or myopathic physiology or valve malfunction when noninvasive imaging and Doppler data are inconclusive, inconsistent, or in conflict with the clinical findings.[4] Hemodynamic assessment can be particularly important for decisions regarding repeat pericardial removal or valve replacement with the inherent increased morbidity and mortality of second or third operations. In valvular cases with either mechanical aortic or aortic and mitral valve

prostheses, transseptal catheterization and direct left ventricular puncture have been used to obtain critical transvalvular hemodynamic data and assess the angiographic severity of the mitral regurgitation.[4]

Planning of the procedure to determine the best opportunities to gather the pressure and flow data before the patient enters the catheterization laboratory is essential. Most cases require an accurate assessment of cardiac output,

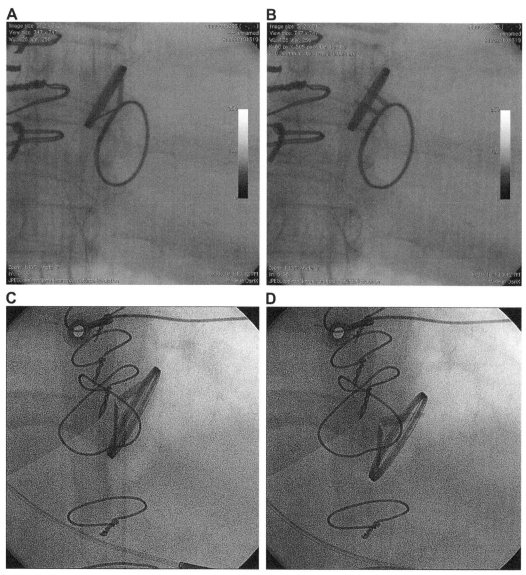

Fig. 3. Cinefluoroscopic images of bileaflet tilting disc mechanical valves. (*A*) A normal-appearing aortic valve with the discs in the closed position. There is a ring enclosing the mitral valve annulus just below the aortic valve. (*B*) The same valve in the open position. As seen in these images, the discs do not quite achieve a 90 degree opening angle, nor do they achieve a flat appearance when closed. (*C*) A mechanical mitral valve imaged in the closed position in a different patient. Note the lack of difference in leaflet position between this image and the one in (*D*), which was obtained during systole at maximum opening of the valve. The patient in (*C*) and (*D*) had restricted movement of one of the leaflets, resulting in a large gradient across the valve.

mandating the performance of a detailed right heart catheterization to obtain thermodilution or Fick estimates of flow. Furthermore, the evaluation of the pressures from the right atrium, right ventricle, pulmonary artery, and pulmonary capillary wedge positions gives insight into the degree of physiologic impairment that may exist secondary to prosthetic valvular dysfunction. Routine measurement of simultaneous pressures on either side of the prosthetic valve should be the hallmark of the invasive hemodynamic

evaluation. Studies have shown the safety of retrograde passage of standard catheters (eg, multipurpose or pigtail) to measure gradients across bioprosthetic and ball-and-cage mechanical valves.[5]

TECHNIQUE OF HIGH-FIDELITY INVASIVE PRESSURE ASSESSMENT

In cases with either mechanical aortic or aortic andmitral valve prostheses, transseptal

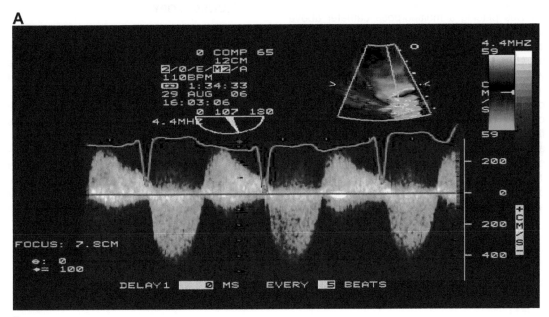

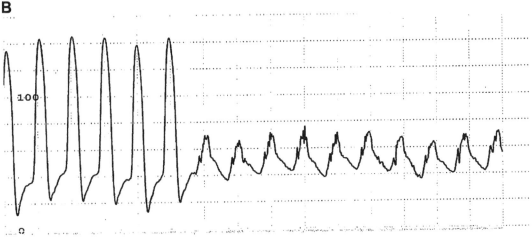

Fig. 4. (*A*) A pullback is performed across the prosthetic valve using a 0.014″ pressure wire. As can be seen on inspection of this pressure tracing, the left ventricular pressure is about 140 mm Hg systolic with an extremely increased end-diastolic pressure (left side of the figure). As the wire is pulled across the aortic valve, a pressure drop of 70 mm Hg is seen. The aortic pressure in this patient is only 70/40 mm Hg. (*B*) A continuous wave Doppler tracing from a simultaneously performed transesophageal echocardiogram shows a similarly increased gradient across the prosthetic valve.

catheterization and direct left ventricular puncture have been used to obtain hemodynamic data and assess the angiographic severity of the mitral regurgitation. Standard retrograde catheter access across mechanical atrioventricular prosthesis has been associated with complications caused by catheter entrapment in the minor valve orifice that may be fatal.[6] To assess the gradient across prosthetic aortic valves, a 0.014" pressure wire can be used to safely cross the valve and directly record the pressure as an alternative to transseptal or apical puncture.[7] The technique involves placing a multipurpose catheter above the aortic valve, followed by the administration of intravenous heparin. Using an angioplasty technique and a Y-connector, a 0.014" pressure guidewire is then advanced to the tip of the multipurpose catheter and the catheter and wire pressures are then equalized identically to the process before performing coronary fractional flow reserve. The guidewire can then be advanced a short distance across the valve and the multipurpose catheter remains above the valve so as not to interfere with valve leaflet mobility. Left ventricular pressure is then obtained from the pressure wire and can be compared with the aortic pressure or

right ventricular pressure (if there is a consideration of pericardial constriction).

Parham and colleagues[8] were able to show that a pressure wire could easily be passed through a #21 St Jude prosthesis (**Fig. 2**). Despite manually forcing the leaflets closed, the guidewire was easily pulled back without resistance. The investigators were unable to find any maneuvers that could produce guidewire entrapment within the valve discs.

CINEFLUOROSCOPY

Cinefluoroscopy provides another means to assess prosthetic valve integrity when acoustic shadowing from the echocardiogram limits the ability to determine normal leaflet functioning and Doppler gradients may be higher than expected (**Fig. 3**). Mechanical valves have a distinctive appearance and proper mobility of the leaflets and or ball-and-cage valve can quickly be judged. Another finding seen via cine involves a characteristic rocking motion that may develop in patients with valvular dehiscence. One major advantage to these images is the lack of need for contrast so patients can quickly be assessed even in the

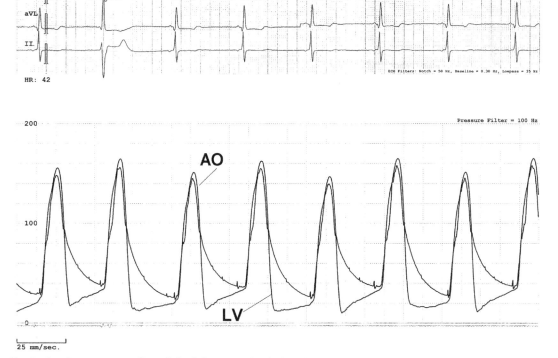

Fig. 5. Simultaneous recording of the left ventricular (LV) and aortic (AO) pressures across a dysfunctional prosthetic aortic valve. As described in the text, the LV pressure is obtained from a 0.014" pressure wire and the AO pressure is obtained through a multipurpose catheter.

setting of acute renal failure or with difficulties in obtaining vascular access. Often, noninvasive cinefluoroscopy can reassure the clinician and the patient to the point that direct measurement of the hemodynamic gradient may not be needed.

CASE EXAMPLES

1. A patient was noted to have a history of Medtronic Hall valve placement in the aortic position approximately 5 years before presenting to the catheterization laboratory with complaints of chest pain with inferolateral ST depression on the electrocardiogram. After the patient was found to have no significant coronary obstruction, fluoroscopy confirmed poor movement of the bileaflet aortic valve. A pressure wire was then advanced and withdrawn through the restricted valve while awaiting transesophageal echocardiogram with the pressure tracing as shown (**Fig. 4**). There was a gradient of approximately 70 mm Hg across the aortic valve. Doppler assessment via transesophageal echocardiogram confirmed a peak gradient of 75 mm Hg. The echo further showed that there was material consistent with thrombus on the valvular leaflets. Cardiac surgical consultation was obtained and deemed the patient to be at high risk for reoperation and the patient was given intravenous thrombolytic therapy.[8,9] Immediate improvement was noted in the valvular function.

2. A complex patient was brought to the catheterization laboratory with significant worsening of shortness of breath in a 4-week period. She had a history of chest radiation for non-Hodgkin lymphoma, with subsequent aortic valve and mitral valve replacement surgery after she was found to have developed aortic stenosis and mitral stenosis, presumably as a complication of the radiation. Several years later, she underwent reoperation to replace her aortic valve, because her first operation was only able to get a 19-mm prosthetic valve

in place and she had shortness of breath that was attributed to a patient–prosthetic valve mismatch. A supravalvular aortic valve was implanted to try to improve her effective prosthetic valve orifice area, and the patient's symptoms were relieved until the present setback. Before catheterization, echocardiography showed a moderate amount of AI and a suggestion of constrictive physiology. As seen in **Fig. 5**, using a multipurpose catheter in the ascending aorta and a pressure wire in the left ventricle, the patient has severe AI with equalization of left ventricular and aortic end-diastolic pressure. In contrast with acute insufficiency, this tracing does not show tachycardia, the end-diastolic pressure is actually high, and the pulse pressure is wide (**Table 3** lists the features that differentiate acute from chronic AI). The patient did not have any signs of constriction on any of her pressure tracings, and therefore was felt to have dyspnea secondary to severe AI.

In conclusion, catheter-based measurements of prosthetic valve hemodynamics remain an important part of the assessment of proper function. Echocardiography has supplanted the need for routine invasive hemodynamic assessment of most mechanical prostheses. However, there are times when invasive hemodynamics are required to confirm clinical suspicions of dysfunctional valves. Although invasive hemodynamics are sometimes difficult to obtain (ie, tilting discs), the technique of using a pressure wire to cross prosthetic aortic valves should be considered as a necessary tool in the catheterization laboratory to obtain accurate measurements. The case examples presented here should encourage operators to gain comfort in the technique of passing a pressure wire across an aortic valve tilting disc valves. However, careful technique with consideration of the quality and accuracy of the hemodynamic tracings remain the hallmarks of good invasive prosthetic valve assessment in the catheterization laboratory.

Table 3
Hemodynamic features of chronic versus acute severe AI

	Acute	Chronic
Left ventricular end-diastolic pressure	Markedly increased	May be normal
Aortic systolic pressure	Normal to decreased	Increased
Aortic diastolic pressure	Normal to decreased	Markedly decreased
Pulse pressure	Slightly increased	Markedly increased

REFERENCES

1. Hufnagel CA, Harvey WP. The surgical correction of aortic regurgitation: preliminary report. Bull Georgetown Univ Med Cent 1953;6:60–1.

2. Bonow RO, Carabello BA, Chatterjee K, et al. 2008 focused update incorporated into the ACC/AHA 2006 guidelines for the management of patients with valvular heart disease: a report of the American College of Cardiology/American Heart Association Task Force on Practice Guidelines (Writing Committee to Develop Guidelines for the Management of Patients with Valvular Heart Disease). J Am Coll Cardiol 2008;52:e1–142.

3. Burstow DJ, Nishimura RA, Bailey KR, et al. Continuous wave Doppler echocardiographic measurements of prosthetic valve gradients. A simultaneous Doppler-catheter correlative study. Circulation 1989; 80:504–14.

4. Knebel F, Gliech V, Walde T, et al. High concordance of invasive and echocardiographic mean pressure gradients in patients with a mechanical aortic valve prosthesis. J Heart Valve Dis 2005;14(3):332–7.

5. Fusman B, Faxon D, Feldman T. Hemodynamic rounds: transvalvular pressure gradient measurement. Catheter Cardiovasc Interv 2001;53:553–61.

6. Hortkotte D. Retrograde catheterization of left ventricle through mechanical aortic prostheses. Eur Heart J 1988;9:194–5.

7. Horstokotte D, Jehle J, Loogen F. Death due to transprosthetic catheterization of a Bjork-Shiley prosthesis in the aortic position. Am J Cardiol 1986;58:566–7.

8. Parham W, El Shafei A, Rajjoub H, et al. Retrograde left ventricular hemodynamic assessment across bileaflet prosthetic aortic valves: the use of a high-fidelity pressure sensor angioplasty guidewire. Catheter Cardiovasc Interv 2003;59:509–13.

9. Nguyen PK, Wassermann SM, Fann JI, et al. Successful lysis of an aortic prosthetic valve thrombosis with a dosing regimen for peripheral artery and bypass graft occlusions. J Thorac Cardiovasc Surg 2008;135:691–3.

Coronary Physiology in the Cath Lab: Beyond the Basics

Morton J. Kern, MD, FSCAI

KEYWORDS

- Coronary artery disease
- Cardiac catheterization laboratory
- Translesional pressure measurement
- In-lab coronary physiology

Treating patients with coronary artery disease (CAD) frequently requires assessment of myocardial ischemia before recommending coronary revascularization. Common clinical practice is to challenge the coronary blood supply, that is, provoke myocardial ischemia by employing any one of several outpatient stress tests. The adequacy of coronary blood flow and freedom from ischemia are indicated by the responses to exercise or pharmacologic stimulation observing the associated electrocardiographic changes, deficits of myocardial perfusion, or failure of the left ventricle to thicken or shorten on echocardiography. In a similar fashion and for similar reasons, the ischemic potential of a stenosis can be assessed in the cardiac catheterization laboratory at the time of angiography using sensor-tipped angioplasty guidewires to measure coronary blood flow and pressure across stenotic artery segments.[1,2] The adoption of invasive coronary physiologic lesion assessment before percutaneous coronary intervention (PCI) has become routine in many catheterization laboratories. Indeed, in the last decade, numerous studies have demonstrated favorable outcomes for revascularization decisions based on in-lab coronary physiology in patients with intermediate single-vessel stenoses,[3,4] bifurcation and ostial branch stenoses,[5,6] multivessel CAD, and left main stenoses.[7–10] The use of coronary physiology in the laboratory has been identified as a class IIa recommendation for patients in whom the clinical presentation and supporting data (ie, angiograms,

stress tests) are too inconclusive to make an objective decision regarding treatment.[11] The following discussion reviews selected pertinent concepts and studies of the more complex applications of translesional pressure measurements for optimal patient outcomes.

RATIONALE FOR IN-LAB CORONARY PHYSIOLOGY

The rationale for use of physiologic lesion assessment at the time of angiography is the necessity to overcome the limitation of the angiographic display of a stenosis. Coronary angiography produces 2-dimensional silhouette images of the 3-dimensional vascular lumen. Customarily in clinical practice, the angiographic stenosis severity is visually assessed as a percent diameter reduction from the ratio of the stenosis "minimal" lumen diameter to the adjacent "normal" reference segment diameter, often in a single projection (**Fig. 1**A). The accuracy of this value depends on the observer's objective skills but also is limited by the inability to identify both "diseased" and "normal" vessel segments, particularly in the setting of diffuse CAD.[12] The correlation between minimal lumen diameter and area with hemodynamic lesion significance is poor.[12] To proceed with revascularization one must know the hemodynamic significance of a lesion and, more importantly, that coronary angiography cannot identify the accurate hemodynamic significance of many coronary stenoses, particularly those between

Division of Cardiology, Long Beach Veterans Administration Hospital, University of California, 101 The City Drive, Orange, Irvine, CA 92866, USA
E-mail address: mkern@uci.edu

Cardiol Clin 29 (2011) 237–267
doi:10.1016/j.ccl.2011.01.001
0733-8651/11/$ – see front matter. Published by Elsevier Inc.

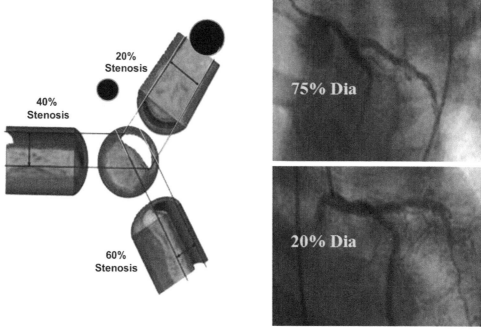

Fig. 1. The rationale for using coronary physiology is the inability of the angiogram to accurately depict lesion characteristics limiting flow. The diagram shows an eccentric lesion, which can be seen as a 20%, 40%, or 60% diameter narrowing from several different angles. This problem is illustrated on the right by the two views of an eccentric left main stem narrowing. The upper image is right anterior oblique projection with caudal angulation; the lower image is right anterior oblique with cranial angulation.

30% and 80% diameter stenosis. This limitation has been documented repeatedly by poor correlation to the variety of stress-testing modalities employed in patients with CAD. Moreover, even sophistical imaging, such as densitometry, rotational angiography, multidetector-row computed tomographic angiography,[13] or 3-dimensional reconstruction, does not reliably reflect the physiologic significance of a given lesion.

CORONARY HEMODYNAMICS

Coronary flow through a normal epicardial artery encounters near zero resistance. As atherosclerosis develops, the altered laminar flow properties as well as obstructing topographic features of a stenosis produce resistance to flow, which is translated as pressure loss due to energy loss (overcoming resistance to flow).[14] The morphologic features of coronary stenosis (ie, shape, length, angulations) responsible for increasing epicardial resistance ultimately limit blood flow and produce angina. Most of these features cannot be accurately discerned from the angiogram. Unlike intravascular ultrasound (IVUS) and computed tomographic angiography, angiography does not provide vascular wall detail sufficient to characterize plaque size, length, and eccentricity.

Moreover, an eccentric angiographic lumen produces conflicting degrees of diameter narrowing when viewed from different radiographic angulations, and introduces uncertainty related to lumen size and its relationship to coronary blood flow. Furthermore, stenosis length and reference vessel diameter play a significant role in the genesis of the pressure gradient across a given stenotic segment. A long moderate narrowing can be as or more hemodynamically significant than a short, focal severe narrowing (**Fig. 2**).[15,16] Angiographic images often include contrast streaming, branch overlap, vessel foreshortening, calcifications, and ostial origins, which further limit the observer's assessment of the stenosis. Given the limitations of the angiogram, the true value of translesional pressure measurements is the incorporation all unknown factors producing resistance and yielding the net distal pressure, to determine the ischemic potential and significance to the patient.

Computation of Pressure-Derived Fractional Flow Reserve

Fractional Flow Reserve (FFR) is derived from the relationship between pressure, flow, and resistance in a coronary artery and corresponding myocardial region. The goal of FFR is to provide

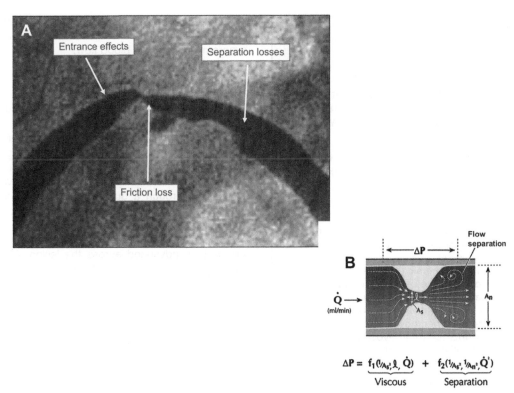

Fig. 2. Factors contributing to pressure loss across a stenosis involve total morphology of the narrowing, not just the most narrowed diameter. Energy loss is produced by friction, separation, and turbulence. Energy is taken out as heat and pressure loss results. The loss of distal pressure is related to the blood flow rate. The angiographic 2-dimensional images cannot account for the multiple factors that produce resistance to coronary blood flow and loss of pressure across a stenosis. The eccentric and irregular stenosis (A) shows arrows designating entrance effects, friction, and zones of turbulence accounting for separation energy loss. The calculation of pressure loss (ΔP) across a stenosis (B) incorporates l = length, A_s = areas stenosis, A_n = reference area, Q = flow, f_1 and f_2 coefficients of viscous friction and laminar separation as contributors to resistance and, hence, pressure loss.

a measurement of the flow (Q) in the stenotic artery as a percentage of normal flow through the same artery in the theoretical absence of the stenosis. FFR is a ratio of flow derived from a ratio of coronary and aortic pressure.[2] The first assumption in the derivation of FFR is that pressure in a normal coronary artery is equal to aortic pressure. The normal left anterior descending artery (LAD) coronary artery pressure is aortic pressure (Pa).

Thus, resistance to flow, R = Q/P (P, pressure);

$$Qs \ = \ Pd/Rd \ \ \text{and} \ \ Qn \ = \ Pa/Ra$$

where *Qs* is stenotic artery flow, *Qn* is normal artery flow, *Pd* is distal coronary pressure, *Pa* is aortic pressure, and *Rd*, *Ra* are the resistances in the myocardial bed beyond the stenosis.

$$FFR \ = \ Qs/QN \ = \ (Pd/Rd)/(Pa/Ra)$$

Rd = Ra at maximal hyperemia (ie, minimal and fixed resistance), and these are cancelled from the equation.

Hence, FFR = Pd Pa, during maximal hyperemia

The full derivation of the FFR calculation also employs venous pressure, Pv, and describes FFR of the collateral circulation using coronary occlusion wedge pressure, Pw, which can be found elsewhere.[2] **Box 1** provides a brief derivation of the 3 most commonly used physiologic parameters measured in the cath lab. FFR is distinguished from direct measurement maximal ratios of coronary blood flow (ie, coronary flow reserve [CFR], the ratio of hyperemic to basal blood flow) in several ways. FFR has a single normal value of 1 because FFR uses aortic pressure as the standard comparator. Recall that epicardial resistance to flow is negligible in the absence of disease. Pa is transmitted completely to the distal artery, making both the numerator and denominator the same value in a normal artery.[16] An FFR value of 0.75 means that the stenotic vessel only provides 75% of the normal expected flow in the theoretical absence of the stenosis. FFR is also specific for the resistance of only the epicardial stenosis. Its derivation excludes the confounding influences of the microcirculation, changes in hemodynamics or contractility.[17] Unlike CFR, FFR is minimally influenced by changes in hemodynamics or other conditions known to alter baseline or maximal hyperemic myocardial blood flow.

MEASUREMENT TECHNIQUE

The methods of translesional pressure measurement have been previously reviewed in detail.[15,16] In brief, following diagnostic angiography in the catheterization laboratory and using a technique identical to that of angioplasty, a 0.014-in pressure sensor angioplasty guidewire is inserted through a guiding catheter and into the target artery. Before crossing the stenosis, the sensor wire's pressure signal is matched to the aortic (guide catheter) pressure. The pressure wire is then advanced across the lesion. Coronary hyperemia is then induced, usually with intravenous or intracoronary adenosine,[18,19] though papaverine, adenosine triphosphate, or selective adenosine 2A agonists has been used as well.[18] The pressure distal to the stenosis (Pd) and aortic pressure (Pa) are continuously recorded. FFR is then calculated as Pd/Pa at maximal hyperemia, the nadir of Pd. An example of FFR is shown on **Fig. 3**A, B. It is important to recognize technical artifacts such as guide catheter clamping that would produce a false-negative FFR (see **Fig. 3**C).[16] **Box 2** is a partial list of reasons why one might encounter a false-negative FFR result.

To assess multiple, sequential lesions or diffuse CAD, the pressure wire is pulled back continuously from the distal to proximal vessel segments during hyperemia induced by an intravenous infusion of adenosine. The pressure pullback curve can demonstrate either an abrupt change in distal pressure across a focal narrowing or the gradual pressure recovery of diffuse disease without focal obstructions.

RADIATION, PROCEDURE TIME, AND CONTRAST USE FOR FFR

FFR may increase the radiation dose, procedural time, and contrast medium after a diagnostic coronary angiogram. Ntalianis and colleagues[20] measured radiation dose (mSv), procedural time (minutes), and contrast medium (mL) In 200 patients (mean age 66 ± 10 years) undergoing diagnostic coronary angiography. FFR was measured in at least one intermediate coronary artery stenosis; 296 stenoses (1.5 ± 0.7 stenoses per patient) were assessed. Hyperemia was achieved by intracoronary (n = 180) or intravenous (n = 20) adenosine. The additional mean radiation dose, procedural time, and contrast medium

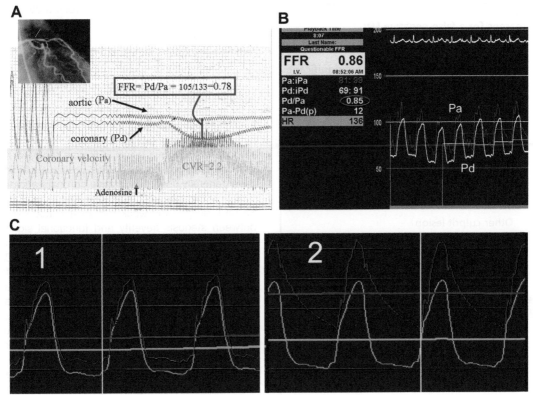

Fig. 3. (*A*) Hemodynamic tracings used to calculate pressure-derived fractional flow reserve (FFR). A mild resting gradient is shown by the difference in the mean aortic and coronary pressures (Pa, Pd), which increases during increasing flow or hyperemia. The hyperemic blood flow signal after adenosine is shown under the yellow shaded band. Coronary vasodilatory reserve, CVR is 2.2 and FFR 0.78. Intracoronary adenosine is indicated by the vertical black arrow. (*B*) Display screen showing FFR pressure signals. Red pressure signal is aortic pressure (Pa) and yellow signal is distal coronary pressure (Pd). In this example, FFR is 0.85. (*C*) Example of pressure signals acquired with deep-seated guide catheter. Guide pressure damping results in matched distal coronary pressure and false-negative FFR value.

needed to obtain FFR as a percentage of the entire procedure were 30% ± 16% (median 4 mSv, range 2.4–6.7 mSv), 26% ± 13% (median 9 minutes, range 7–13 minutes), and 31% ± 16% (median 50 mL, range 30–90 mL), respectively, The procedural time was slightly longer with intravenous adenosine (median 11 minutes vs 9 minutes, *P* = .04). There was no difference between intravenous and intracoronary adenosine for radiation or contrast dosages (**Fig. 4**). There was no difference between intravenous and intracoronary adenosine. When FFR was measured in 3 or more lesions, radiation dose, procedural time, and contrast medium increased. The minimal increases in radiation dose, procedural time, and contrast medium were low compared with IVUS or angioscopy. The clinical value of FFR measurements is worth the small additional radiation and procedure time involved.

FFR THRESHOLD OF ISCHEMIA

FFR values of less than 0.75 are associated with abnormal stress testing results in numerous comparative studies.[21] FFR values greater than 0.80 are associated with negative ischemic results with a predictive accuracy of 95%. Because of variations in testing techniques and patient subgroups, a small zone of FFR uncertainty (0.75–0.80) with regard to stress testing exists. FFR values falling within the gray zone require additional clinical context for decision making. Given the variances of sensitivity, specificity, positive and negative predictive accuracy among patients, and types of stress testing, it is not surprising that, unlike the initial validation study comparing FFR to 3 different stress tests in the same patient before and after PCI,[1] meta-analysis showed only modest concordance of

Box 2
Reasons for a false-negative FFR

Physiologic Explanations

Stenosis hemodynamically nonsignificant despite angiographic appearance

Small perfusion territory, old myocardial infarction (MI), little viable tissue, small vessel

Abundant collaterals

Severe microvascular disease (rarely affecting FFR)

Interpretable Explanations

Other culprit lesion

Diffuse disease not focal stenosis

Chest pain of noncardiac origin

Technical Explanations

Insufficient hyperemia

Guiding catheter related pitfall (deep engagement, small ostium, side holes)

Electrical drift

Actual False-Negative FFR

Acute phase of ST elevation myocardial infarction

Severe left ventricular hypertrophy

Exercise-induced spasm

Data from Koolen JJ, Pijls NH. Coronary pressure never lies. Catheter Cardiovasc Interv 2008;72:248.

FFR with noninvasive imaging tests.[22] The selection of a clinical "gold standard" of ischemia is a significant limitation for all modalities used to correlate ischemic symptoms with coronary anatomy. The false-positive and false-negative test results of stress studies in patients with multivessel CAD are problematic to use as any singe test as a gold standard. However, given the validation study for single-vessel disease by Pijls and colleagues,[1] in contrast to noninvasive tests, FFR is a more vessel-specific index of the ischemic potential of a lesion. **Table 1** is a summary of important validation studies of FFR.

There remains a theoretical concern that the microcirculation adversely limits the value of FFR.[14] The uncertainty of the microcirculatory contribution to an abnormal FFR can be overcome by combined pressure and flow data such as HSR and microvascular assessment such as index of microcirculatory resistance (IMR) and hyperemic myocardial resistance (HMR).[23–25] Defined as the

hyperemic change in pressure across a stenosis divided by the hyperemic distal velocity, HSR may have better predictive value than FFR for detecting noninvasive ischemia.[23]

VALIDATION OF MAGNETIC RESONANCE IMAGING PERFUSION WITH FFR

Validation of magnetic resonance myocardial perfusion imaging (MRMPI) to detect reversible myocardial ischemia using FFR was reported by Watkins and colleagues.[26] The previous studies have generally used quantitative coronary angiography as the standard to assess the accuracy of MRMPI, despite the weak relationship that exists between stenosis severity and functional significance. To address this limitation of prior validation studies, Watkins and colleagues[26] studied 103 patients undergoing evaluation of angina with MRMPI with stress imaging using intravenous adenosine (140 μg/kg/min), and first-pass 0.1 mmol/kg gadolinium bolus imaging technique to FFR performed within 1 week of MRMPI. Perfusion defects were identified in 121 of 300 coronary artery segments (40%), of which 110 had an FFR less than 0.75; 168 of 179 normally perfused segments had an FFR greater than 0.75. The sensitivity and specificity of MRMPI for the detection of functionally significant coronary stenoses were 91% and 94%, respectively, with positive and negative predictive values of 91% and 94%. It appears that MRMPI can detect functionally significant coronary heart disease with high sensitivity, specificity, and positive and negative predictive values using FFR as the standard.

Melikian and colleagues[27] reported on the correlation between ischemic myocardial perfusion imaging (MPI) with single-photon emission computed tomography (SPECT) with FFR in patients with multivessel coronary disease. Sixty-seven patients (201 vascular territories) with angiographic 2- or 3-vessel coronary disease prospectively underwent MPI (rest/stress adenosine), and FFR in each vessel was measured within 2 weeks. In 42% of patients, MPI and FFR detected identical ischemic territories (mean number of territories 0.9 ± 0.8 for both; $P = 1.00$). In the remaining 36% MPI underestimated (mean number of territories; MPI: 0.46 ± 0.6, FFR: 2.0 ± 0.6; $P<.001$) and in 22% overestimated (mean number of territories; MPI: 1.9 ± 0.8, FFR: 0.5 ± 0.8; $P<.001$) the number of ischemic territories in comparison with FFR. There was poor concordance in detecting myocardial ischemia on both a per-patient ($\kappa = 0.14$ [95% confidence interval: −0.10–0.39]) and per-vessel ($\kappa = 0.28$ [95% confidence interval: 0.15–0.42]) basis. In this study there was poor concordance

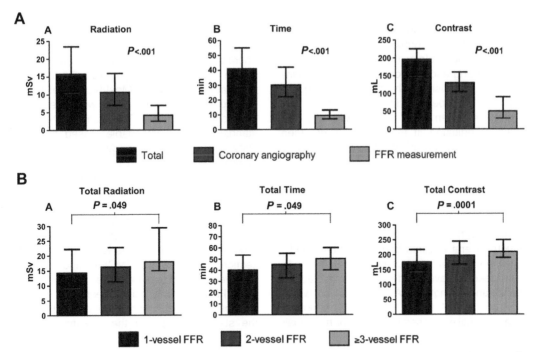

Fig. 4. (*A*) Additional amount of radiation (A), procedure time (B), and contrast medium (C) needed to perform FFR as a percentage of diagnostic and PCI procedure. (*B*) Incremental additional radiation (A), procedure time (B), and contrast medium (C) needed for 1-, 2-, and 3-vessel FFR. (*From* Ntalianis A, Trana C, Muller O, et al. Effective radiation dose, time, and contrast medium to measure fractional flow reserve. J Am Coll Cardiol Interv 2010;3:821–7; with permission.)

of MPI with FFR. MPI tends to under- or overestimate the functional significance of angiographic compared with FFR in patients with multivessel disease.

FFR and IVUS

Confusion and controversy has arisen among some operators presuming that a single minimal lumen area by IVUS can replace the physiologic

Table 1
FFR and noninvasive stress test results

Index	References	Refs.#	N	Ischemic Test	BCV	Acc %
FFR	Pijls	2	60	X-ECG	0.74	97
	DeBruyne	17	60	X-ECG/SPECT	0.72	85
	Pijls	1	45	X-ECG/SPECT/pacing/DSE	0.75	93
	Bartunek	55	37	DSE	0.68	90
	Abe	56	46	SPECT	0.75	91
	Chamuleau	57	127	SPECT	0.74	77
	Caymaz	58	40	SPECT	0.76	95
	Jimenez-Navarro	59	21	DSE	0.75	90
	Usu	60	167	SPECT	0.75	79
	Yanagisawa	61	167	SPECT	0.75	76
	Meuwissen	23	151	SPECT	0.74	85
	DeBruyne	42	57	MIBI-SPECT post MI	0.78	85
	Samady	44	48	MIBI-SPECT post MI	0.78	85
H-SRv	Meuwissen	23	151	SPECT	0.80	87

Abbreviations: Acc%, percent accuracy; BVC, best cut-off value (defined as the value with the highest sum of sensitivity and specificity); DSE, dobutamine stress echocardiography; N, number; SPECT, single-photon emission tomography; X-ECG, exercise electrocardiography.

Modified from Kern MJ, Samady H. Current concepts of integrated coronary physiology in the cath lab. J Am Coll Cardiol 2010;55:173–85; with permission.

measurement of FFR.[28] FFR is designed for physiologic epicardial lesion assessment. IVUS is designed to assess coronary lesion and vessel anatomy and morphology. IVUS is highly accurate for vessel sizing and for confirming stent expansion and strut apposition. The clinician's first question should be "does this lesion limit blood flow and produce ischemia?" If the answer is yes, the stenting is indicated. If the answer is no, then stenting is of no value and introduces unnecessary risk and cost.

There are several IVUS studies that have compared FFR to IVUS measurements such as minimal lumen area (MLA). Tagaki and colleagues[29] found that most MLA values of less than 4 mm² were associated with an FFR of less than 0.75 (**Fig. 5**), although several patients had nonischemic FFR. The reason for this variance is that resistance to flow is based on several different anatomic factors (entrance angle, length, MLA, eccentricity) of which MLA is only one. A 4-mm² MLA may limit flow in a large proximal vessel segments but will not impair flow in a smaller segment of the same artery. Moreover, for left main assessment, unlike FFR, the IVUS threshold for treatment or no treatment changes. There are several different IVUS MLAs reported to be the cut-off value, ranging from 5.9 to 7.0 mm² for treatment decisions. Most IVUS thresholds are derived from clinical outcomes, with different areas from different studies. This variable IVUS "gold standard" is understandable, based on what is known about using only one dimension of a complex stenosis, with or without including the reference vessel segment dimensions. The loss of pressure across a stenosis can be computed from the simplified Bernoulli principle, which includes not only the stenosis area but also the length of the narrowing. $\Delta P = 1/As * length * V^2$, where ΔP is the pressure drop across a stenosis, As is the minimal cross-sectional stenosis area (MCSa), and V is blood flow velocity through the tube. Moreover, unlike IVUS, FFR is not only lesion-specific but also incorporates the variable myocardial blood flow across the stenosis supplying the specific myocardial

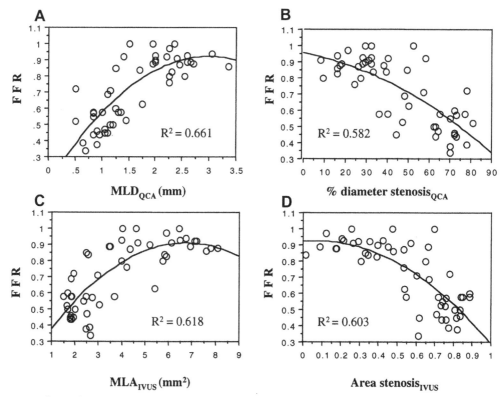

Fig. 5. Correlation between FFR and quantitative coronary angiography and IVUS measurements. (A), FFR vs minimum lumen diameter (MLD) by quantitative coronary angiography (QCA), (B), percent diameter, (C), minimum lumen area (MLA) by IVUSl, (D), area stenosis by IVUS. (*From* Takagi A, Tsurumi Y, Ishii Y, et al. Clinical potential of intravascular ultrasound for physiological assessment of coronary stenosis. Relationship between quantitative ultrasound tomography and pressure-derived fractional flow reserve. Circulation 1999;100:250–5; with permission.)

bed. For example, a 70% stenosis in a vessel sub-tending a small diagonal or a previously infarcted mid-anterior descending territory will have less physiologic impact than an *identical* lesion in a mid-anterior descending subtending a normal anterior wall region because of the significantly higher flow requirements. Iqbal and colleagues[30] demonstrated the dramatic change in the LAD FFR after recanalization of an occluded right coronary artery which was previously supplied by the LAD collateral flow (**Fig 6**). Thus, the FFR will be lower, even though the stenosis dimensions are identical.

The area of a normal 2.5-mm vessel is 4.9 mm². Thus, a stenosis with MLA of 4 mm² (a 28% area stenosis) in this vessel should not be considered obstructive or in need of PCI. Functionally

significant coronary lesions must be greater than 50% diameter stenosis (approximately 75% area stenosis). A coronary narrowing with MLA of 4.0 mm² in a 3.0-mm vessel (area of 7.1 mm²) yields a 44% area stenosis, again questionably associated with ischemia. However, deferring PCI in a lesion with an IVUS-defined MLA greater than 4 mm² is associated with excellent clinical outcome.[31] Several studies[32] demonstrated the poor relationship between FFR and IVUS minimal lesion area (r^2 between 0.4 and 0.6).

Most recently, Nam and colleagues[33] evaluated the long-term clinical outcomes of two strategies of PCI, comparing an FFR-guided PCI strategy with IVUS-guided PCI for intermediate coronary lesions in 167 consecutive patients (FFR-guided, 83 lesions vs IVUS-guided, 94 lesions). Cut-off

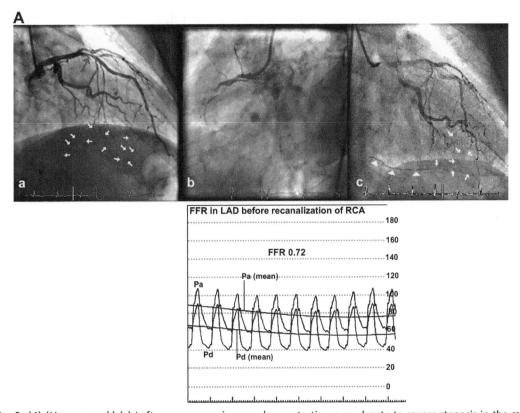

Fig. 6. (*A*) (*Upper panels*) (a) Left coronary angiogram demonstrating a moderate-to-severe stenosis in the mid LAD (*arrow*). Collateral connections from the septal branches of the LAD can be seen (*white arrows*). (b) Right coronary angiogram demonstrating a chronic total occlusion of the right coronary artery (RCA). (c) Late filling of posterior descending artery from retrograde filling (*white arrowheads*) following left coronary injection. (*Lower panel*) FFR of LAD at this time is 0.72. (*B*) The RCA was then approached and successfully recanalized. (*Upper panels*) (a) LAD lesion unchanged angiographically. (b) RCA is now patent after stenting. (c) Collaterals are no longer visible. (*Lower panel*) Repeat FFR of LAD is now 0.84, above the ischemic threshold. (*C*) Illustration of changes in supply bed influencing FFR after RCA recanalization. Because the supply bed of the LAD is markedly reduced after RCA recanalization, the FFR increased from 0.72 to 0.84, demonstrating role of flow on FFR-related ischemic potential. (*From* Iqbal MB, Shah N, Khan M, et al. Reduction in myocardial perfusion territory and its effect on the physiological severity of a coronary stenosis. Circ Cardiovasc Interv 2010;3:89–90; with permission.)

B

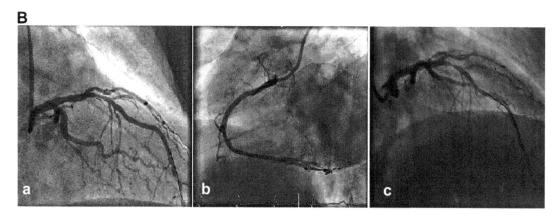

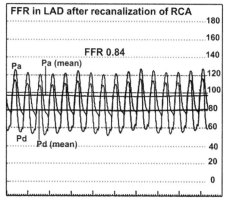

C

LCA perfusion territory prior to recanalization of RCA

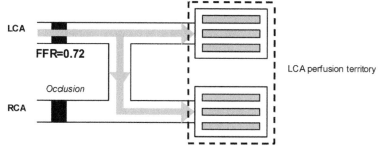

LCA perfusion territory after to recanalization of RCA

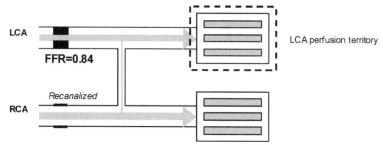

Fig. 6. *(continued)*

value for FFR-guided PCI was 0.80, and for IVUS-guided PCI was a minimal lumen cross-sectional area of 4.0 mm². The initial percent diameter stenosis and lesion length were similar in both groups (51% ± 8% and 24 ± 12 mm in the FFR group vs 52% ± 8% and 24 ± 13 mm in the IVUS group, respectively). However, the IVUS-guided group underwent stenting significantly more often (91.5% vs 33.7%, P<.001) with no significant difference in rates of major adverse cardiac events (MACE) between the two groups (3.6% vs 3.2% in FFR-guided and IVUS-guided PCI, respectively) (**Fig. 7**). Independent predictors for performing intervention were guiding device: FFR versus IVUS (relative risk [RR]: 0.02); artery location: LAD versus non-LAD disease (RR: 5.60); and multi- versus single-vessel disease (RR: 3.28). Although both FFR- and IVUS-guided PCI strategies for intermediate CAD were associated with favorable outcomes, the FFR-guided PCI reduces the need for revascularization of many of these lesions. The health care economic implications of this comparison are self evident.

CLINICAL APPLICATIONS OF FFR FOR DIFFICULT ANGIOGRAPHIC SUBSETS
Intermediate Lesions and the Patient with Multivessel CAD

Many patients may have multivessel CAD with at least one obviously severe lesion and others that are intermediately narrowed (30%–80%). Using FFR for revascularization decisions for such lesions has demonstrated excellent long-term results. The DEFER study[4] randomized 325 patients scheduled for PCI into 3 groups and reported the 5-year outcomes. Patients were

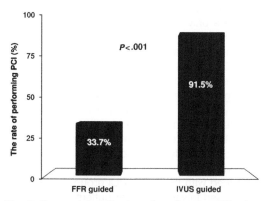

Fig. 7. Comparison of rates of performing PCI when guided by FFR or IVUS. (*From* Nam CW, Yoon HJ, Cho YK, et al. Outcomes of percutaneous coronary intervention in intermediate coronary artery disease: fractional flow reserve–guided versus intravascular ultrasound guided. J Am Coll Cardiol Interv 2010;3:812–7; with permission.)

randomly assigned to the deferral group (n = 91), If FFR was 0.75 or greater, with continued medical therapy or the PCI performance group (n = 90, PCI with stents). If FFR was less than 0.75, PCI was performed as planned and patients were entered into the reference group (n = 144). Overall, the event-free survival was not different between the deferred and performed group (80% and 73% respectively, P = .52), and both were significantly better than in the reference group (63%, P = .03). The composite rate of cardiac death and acute MI in the deferred, performed, and reference groups was 3.3%, 7.9%, and 15.7%, respectively (P = .21 for deferred vs performed and P = .003 for reference vs both of the deferred and performed groups) (**Fig. 8**). The percentage of patients free from chest pain on follow-up was not different between the deferred and performed groups. The 5-year risk of cardiac death or MI in patients with normal FFR is less than 1% per year and was not decreased by stenting. Treating patients with intermediate lesions assisted by FFR is associated with a low event rate, comparable to event rates in patients with normal noninvasive testing. Similar outcomes for deferment of lesions with FFR greater than 0.80 is also reported in patients undergoing multivessel revascularization guided by FFR.[7,34,35]

FFR-Guided Multivessel PCI

One of the large confounders in the assessment and management of patients with multivessel disease is the uncertainty of ischemia related to a specific lesion. It is now known that not all multivessel angiographic CAD is physiologically equivalent CAD. This counterintuitive phenomenon has been demonstrated by Tonino and colleagues,[36] who assessed FFR in all 3 vessels in patients with multivessel CAD. The incidence of "significant" 3-vessel angiographic CAD dropped from 27% to 9%, 2-vessel CAD dropped from 43% to 17%, and single-vessel disease increased from 30% to 60%. Most recently Tonino and colleagues,[34] in the FAME (FFR vs Angiography for Multivessel Evaluation) study 2-year follow-up, also demonstrated the striking difference between anatomic and physiologic multivessel disease. Before FFR measurements, at the time of randomization into the study, of the total 1329 lesions that were successfully assessed by the FFR, angiographic lesions were grouped by severity into 3 categories: 50% to 70% (47% of all lesions), 71% to 90% (39% of all lesions), and 91% to 99% (15% of all lesions) diameter stenosis by visual assessment. In the category 50% to 70% stenosis, 35% were functionally significant (FFR <0.80) and 65% were not (FFR >0.80)

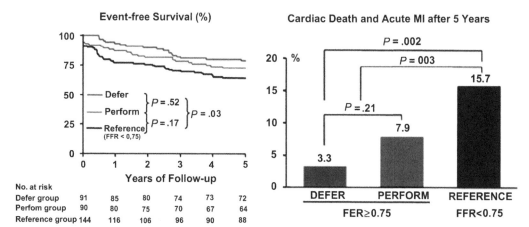

Fig. 8. Five-year follow-up from the DEFER Study. (*Left panel*) Event-free survival curves for the Defer, Perform, and Reference groups. (*Right panel*) Incidence of cardiac death/MI for the 3 groups. (*From* Pijls NH, Van Schaardenburgh P, Manoharan G, et al. Percutaneous coronary intervention of functionally non-significant stenoses: 5-year follow-up of the DEFER study. J Am Coll Cardiol 2007;49:2105–11; with permission.)

(Fig. 9). In the category 71% to 90% stenosis, 80% were functionally significant and 20% were not. In the category 91% to 99% stenosis, 96% were functionally significant. Of all 509 patients with angiographically defined multivessel disease, only 235 (46%) had functional multivessel disease (>2 coronary arteries with an FFR <0.80). This analysis demonstrated that angiography continues to be inaccurate in assessing the functional significance of a coronary stenosis when compared with the FFR, not only in the 50% to 70% angiographic severity category but also in the 70% to 90% category. The reduction in the number of vessels that are physiologically significant has an impact on selection of patients for the different available revascularization options.

Both nonrandomized and prospective randomized studies demonstrated the benefit of FFR guidance in patients with multivessel CAD. Berger and colleagues[8] showed a reduction in MACE in 102 patients with multivessel CAD with planned PCI of at least 2 vessels. In 113 coronary arteries with baseline FFR of 0.57 ± 0.13, PCI was performed and in 127 coronary arteries with an FFR greater than 0.75 (FFR 0.86 ± 0.06), PCI was not performed. Overall, MACE occurred in 9% of patients after 12 months and 13% after 36 months. In the nontreated vessels, 8 (6.3%) MACE were reported whereas 14 (12.3%) MACE were related to one of the initially PCI-treated coronary arteries. Similarly, FFR-guided PCI (FFR-PCI) was compared with angiographically guided PCI (Angio-PCI) in 137 patients with multivessel CAD.[9] Compared with the FFR-PCI group, there were more vessels per patient treated in the Angio-PCI group (2.27 ± 0.50 vs 1.12 ± 0.30 vessels) at a higher cost ($3167 ± $1194 vs $2572 ± $934, respectively; P<.001). The 30-month Kaplan-Meier event-free survival was significantly higher in the FFR-PCI group than in the Angio-PCI group (89% vs 59%, P<.01).

The largest prospective randomized, multicenter trial showing the benefit of this approach was the FAME trial.[7,34,35] Tonino and colleagues[34] compared a physiologically guided PCI approach (FFR-PCI) with a conventional angiographically guided PCI (Angio-PCI) in patients with multivessel CAD. Twenty centers in Europe and the United States randomly assigned 1005 patients with multivessel CAD undergoing PCI with drug-eluting stents to one of the two strategies. Operators selected all indicated lesions in advance of randomization for stenting by visual angiographic appearance (>50% diameter stenosis). For the FFR-PCI group, all lesions had FFR measurements and were only stented if the FFR was less than 0.80. Of the 1005 patients, 496 were assigned to the Angio-PCI and 509 were assigned to the FFR-PCI. Clinical characteristics and angiographic findings were similar in both groups. The Syntax (Synergy between PCI with Taxus and Cardiac Surgery) scores for gauging risk in multivessel disease involvement were identical at 14.5, indicating low- to intermediate-risk patients.

Despite identifying in advance 3 angiographically indicated lesions per patient for stenting, compared with the Angio-PCI group the FFR-PCI group used fewer stents per patient (1.9 ± 1.3 vs 2.7 ± 1.2, P<.001), less contrast medium (272 mL vs 302 mL, P<.001), had lower procedure cost ($5332 vs $6007, P<.001), and shorter hospital stay (3.4 vs 3.7 days, P = .05). More importantly, at 1 year follow-up the FFR-PCI group had fewer MACE (13.2% vs 18.4%, P = .02), fewer

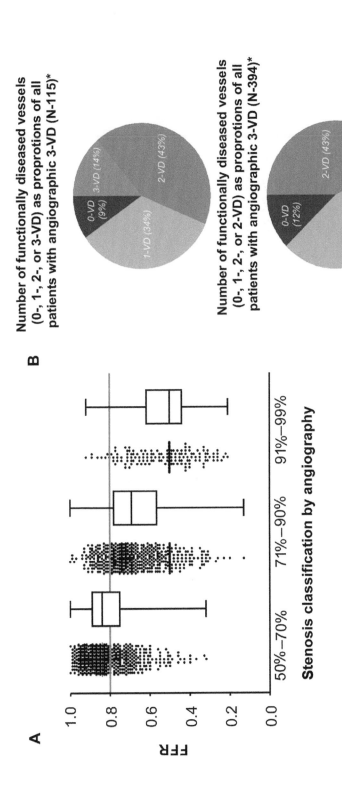

Fig. 9. (*A*) Angiographic severity versus functional severity of coronary artery stenoses by stenosis category. (*B*) Proportions of functionally diseased coronary arteries in patients with angiographic (*upper*) 3- or (*lower*) 2-vessel disease. (*From* Tonino PA, Fearon WF, De Bruyne B, et al. Angiographic versus functional severity of coronary artery stenoses in the fame study, fractional flow reserve versus angiography in multivessel evaluation. J Am Coll Cardiol 2010;55:2816–21; with permission.)

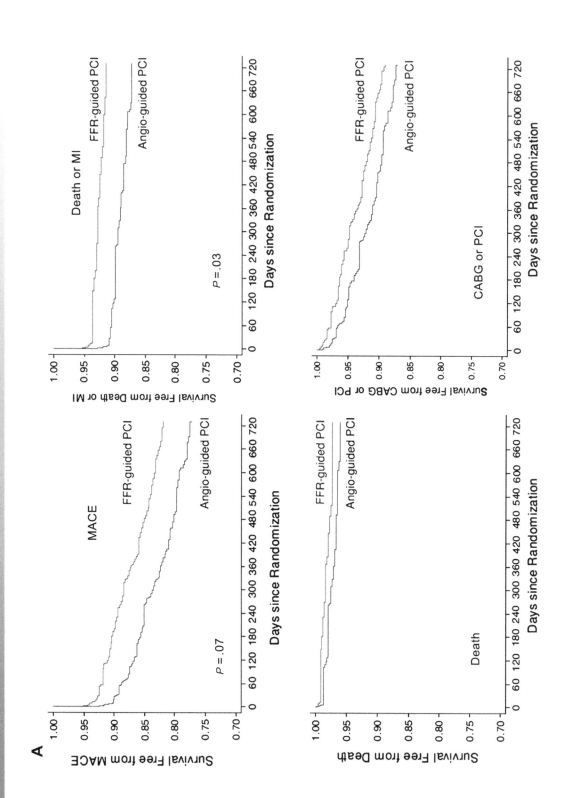

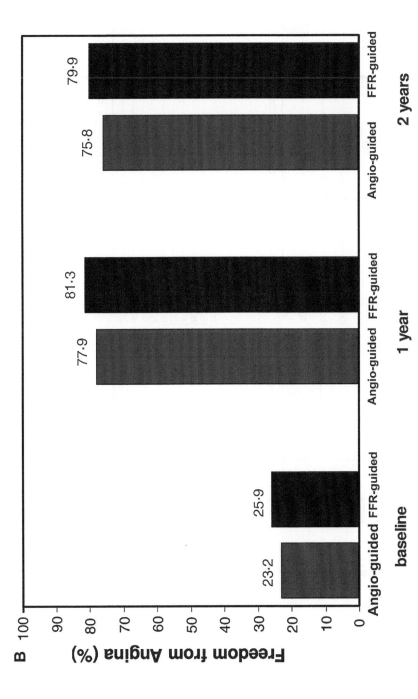

Fig. 10. (*A*) Two-year outcome of stenoses in FFR group initially deferred on basis of FFR >0.80. Numbers of late myocardial infarction and repeat revascularization of the stenoses in the FFR group initially deferred from stenting on the basis of FFR >0.80, and in stenoses in the FFR group that were stented because of FFR 0.80. (*B*) Percentage of patients treated by angiography-guided strategy (*red bars*) and fractional flow reserve (FFR)-guided strategy (*blue bars*) who were completely free from angina at baseline, and at 1- and 2-year follow-up. CABG, coronary artery bypass grafting; MACE, major adverse cardiac event. (*From* Pijls NH, Fearon WF, Tonino PA, et al. Fractional flow reserve versus angiography for guiding percutaneous coronary intervention in patients with multivessel coronary artery disease: 2-year follow-up of the FAME (Fractional Flow Reserve Versus Angiography for Multivessel Evaluation) study. J Am Coll Cardiol 2010;56:177–84; with permission.)

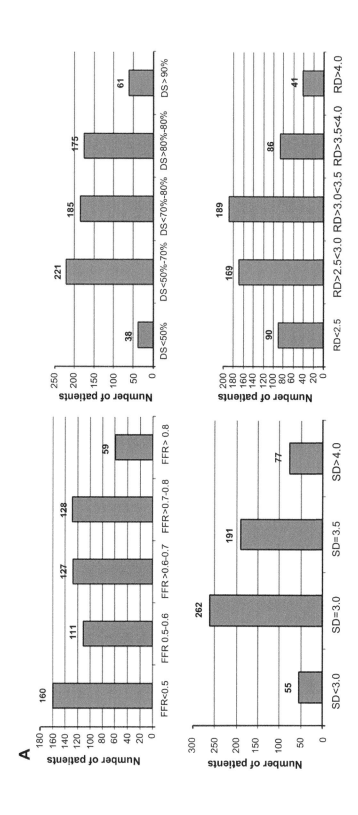

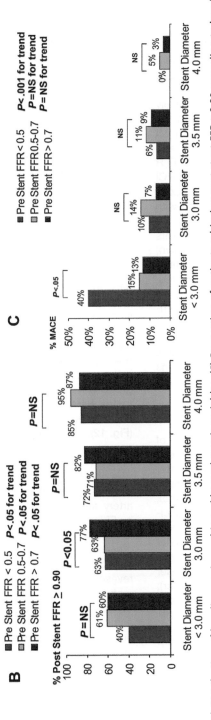

Fig. 11. (A) Distribution of baseline angiographic and hemodynamic variables. (B) Proportion of patients achieving post-stent FFR ≥0.90 according to baseline FFR and stent diameter. (C) Incidence of MACE rates according to SD and baseline FFR. (*From* Samady H, McDaniel M, Veledar E, et al. Baseline fractional flow reserve and stent diameter predict optimal post-stent fractional flow reserve and major adverse cardiac events after bare-metal stent deployment. J Am Coll Cardiol Interv 2009;2:357–63; with permission.)

combined death or MI (7.3% vs 11%, $P = .04$), and a lower total number of MACE including death, MI, and repeat revascularization (coronary artery bypass grafting [CABG] or PCI) (76 vs 113, $P = .02$) than the Angio-PCI group. The 2-year rates of mortality or MI from the FAME study[7] were 12.9% in the angiography-guided group and 8.4% in the FFR-guided group ($P = .02$). Rates of PCI or coronary artery bypass surgery were 12.7% and 10.6%, respectively ($P = .30$). Combined rates of death, nonfatal MI, and revascularization were 22.4% and 17.9%, respectively ($P = .08$) (**Fig. 10**). For lesions deferred on the basis of FFR greater than 0.80, the rate of MI was 0.2% and the rate of revascularization was 3.2% after 2 years. Routine measurement of FFR in patients with multivessel CAD undergoing PCI with drug-eluting stents significantly reduces mortality and MI at 2 years when compared with standard angiography-guided PCI.

The precise mechanisms of reduced end points in the FFR-guided arm of FAME are not known, but are likely associated with fewer implanted stents having fewer procedure-related early (eg, side branch occlusion, additional troponin release) and late stent complications (eg, subacute thrombosis, restenosis). This study is a substantial clinical validation of the preceding FFR outcome studies in single- and multivessel-disease patients from single centers, and has important implications for managing CAD patients by integrating physiology for best long-term results.

FFR and outcome of stenting

Samady and colleagues[37] reported on the use of FFR to predict post-stent MACE after bare metal stent (BMS) in 586 patients from the multicenter post-BMS FFR registry. Multivariable logistic regression models were used to identify clinical, angiographic, and hemodynamic variables associated with post-stent FFR of 0.90 or greater and 6-month MACE. Baseline FFR and stent diameter were predictive of post-stent FFR greater than 0.90. Lower FFR (odds ratio [OR]: 7.8); smaller stent diameter (OR: 3.7 per millimeter); longer stent length (OR: 1.0 per millimeter); and larger minimal luminal diameter (OR: 2.2 per millimeter) were predictors of MACE. In patients receiving 3-mm diameter stents, baseline FFR greater than 0.70 yielded significantly higher likelihood of achieving post-stent FFR greater than 0.90 than baseline FFR 0.70 or less (77% vs 63%, $P<.05$); and in patients receiving stents of diameter less than 3 mm, baseline FFR less than 0.50 was associated with higher MACE than FFR 0.50 to 0.70 and FFR greater than 0.70 (40% vs 15% vs 13%, $P<.05$) (**Fig. 11**). These variables

may allow selection of patients who will have excellent results with BMS.

Assessment of Left Main Stenosis

Correct clinical assessment left main stem CAD lesions is of critical importance to patients facing possible CABG surgery or medical therapy. On the basis of angiographic information alone, this evaluation often cannot be done reliably. FFR can support decision making in equivocal left main disease. In prospective single-center studies, Bech and colleagues[9] and others (**Table 2**) found that consecutive patients with intermediate left main coronary artery stenosis (42% ± 13% diameter) and FFR greater than 0.80 did as well when treated medically as those patients with FFR of less than 0.75 who underwent CABG. MACE at 14 months follow-up was 13% and 7%, respectively ($P = .27$); cardiac death or MI was also similar (6% and 7%, $P = .70$).

In a larger multicenter prospective trial, Hamilos and colleagues[10] examined FFR in 213 patients with an angiographically equivocal left main coronary artery stenosis, When FFR was greater than 0.80, patients were treated medically or another stenosis was treated by coronary angioplasty (nonsurgical group; n = 138). When FFR was less than 0.80, CABG was performed (surgical group; n = 75). The 5-year survival estimates were 89.8% in the nonsurgical group and 85.4% in the surgical group ($P = .48$). The 5-year event-free survival estimates were 74.2% and 82.8% in the nonsurgical and surgical groups, respectively ($P = .50$) (**Fig. 12**). Percent diameter stenosis at quantitative coronary angiography correlated significantly with FFR ($r = 0.38$, $P<.001$), but a very large scatter was observed. In 23% of patients with a diameter stenosis greater than 50%, the left main coronary artery stenosis was hemodynamically significant by FFR. In patients with equivocal stenosis of the left main coronary artery, angiography does not correlate with functional significance. Erroneous individual decision making about the need for revascularization may occur that relies on angiography alone (see **Table 2**). The role of IVUS should be carefully evaluated because of the unaccounted anatomic factors involved.[10] The favorable outcomes suggest that FFR should be assessed in equivocal left main patients before finalizing a revascularization decision.

Ostial Lesion and Side Branch Assessment

Ostial narrowings of side branches or newly produced narrowing in side branches within stents (called "jailed" branches) are difficult to assess by angiography because of the overlapping

Table 2
FFR to assess intermediate left main coronary disease

Study	References	FFR Threshold	N	Medical Therapy			Surgical Therapy			Follow-up Time (mo)
				N (%)	MACE	Death	N (%)	MACE	Death	
Hamilos (2009)	10	0.8	213	136 (65%)	26%	9 (6.5%)	73 (35%)	17%	7 (9.6%)	35 ± 25
Courtis (2009)	62	0.75 surg 0.80 med	142	82 (58%)	13%	3 (3.6%)	60 (42%)	7%	3 (5%)	14 ± 11
Lindstraedt (2006)	63	0.75 surg 0.80 med	51	24 (47%)	31%	0	27 (53%)	34%	5 (19%)	29 ± 16
Suemaru (2005)	64	0.75	15	8 (53%)	0	0	7 (47%)	29%	0	33 ± 10
Legutko (2005)	65	0.75	38	20 (53%)	10%	0	18 (46%)	11%	2	24, mean
Jimenez-Navarro (2004)	66	0.75	27	20 (74%)	10%	0	7 (26%)	29%	2	2 ± 12
Bech (2001)	9	0.75	54	24 (44%)	24%	0	30 (56%)	17%	1	29 ± 15

Data from Lokhandwala J, Hodgson JB. Assessing intermediate left main lesions with IVUS or FFR. How intravascular ultrasound and fractional flow reserve can be used in this challenging subset. Cardiac Interventions Today 2009. p. 47–58.

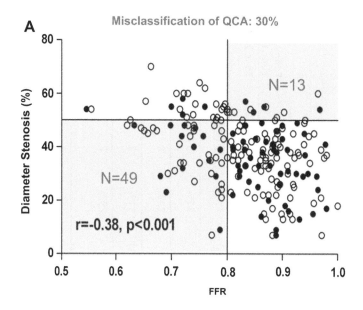

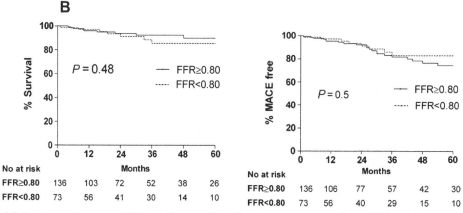

Fig. 12. (*A*) Angiography versus FFR in patients with left main artery narrowings. (*B*) Survival curves for FFR-guided (FFR >0.80) and CABG (FFR <0.80)-treated patients over 5 years. QCA, quantitative coronary angiography. (*B, From* Hamilos M, Muller O, Cuisset T, et al. Long-term clinical outcome after fractional flow reserve–guided treatment in patients with angiographically equivocal left main coronary artery stenosis. Circulation 2009;120:1505–12; with permission.)

orientation relative to the parent branch, stent struts across the branch, and image foreshortening. Koo and colleagues[5,38] compared FFR with quantitative coronary angiography in 97 jailed side branch lesions (vessel size >2.0 mm, percent stenosis >50% by visual estimation) after stent implantation. No lesion with less than 75% stenosis had FFR less than 0.75. Among 73 lesions with 75% or more stenosis, only 20 lesions (27%) were functionally significant. Koo and colleagues[38] also reported the 9-month outcome of FFR-guided side branch PCI strategy for bifurcation lesions. Of 91 patients, side branch intervention was

performed in 26 of 28 patients with FFR less than 0.75. In this subgroup FFR increased to greater than 0.75 despite residual stenosis of 69% ± 10%. At 9 months, functional restenosis was 8% (5/65) with no difference in events compared with 110 side branches treated by angiography alone (4.6% vs 3.7%, P = .7) (**Fig. 13**). Measurement of FFR for ostial and side branch assessment identifies the minority of lesions that are functionally significant.

Koo and colleagues[39] also evaluated the anatomic physiology of the bifurcation lesion to identify the predictors of functionally significant

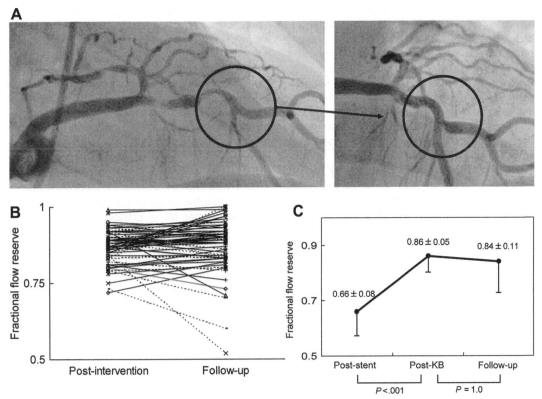

Fig. 13. (*A*) Example of PCI with newly jailed side branch. (*B*) Changes of fractional flow reserve in each lesion (*solid line*: no kissing balloon inflation; *dotted line*: kissing balloon inflation). (*C*) Serial changes of fractional flow reserve in 22 lesions with kissing balloon inflation (KB). (*C, From* Koo BK, Park KW, Kang HJ, et al. Physiologic evaluation of the provisional side-branch intervention strategy for bifurcation lesions using fractional flow reserve. Eur Heart J 2008;29(6):726–32; with permission.)

jailed side branch lesions in 77 patients from 8 centers. Main branch IVUS was performed before and after main branch stenting and FFR was measured in the jailed side branch. The vessel volume index of both the proximal and distal main branch was increased after stent implantation. The plaque volume index decreased in the proximal main branch (9.1 ± 3.0 to 8.4 ± 2.4 mm³/mm, P = .001) implicating plaque shift, but not in the distal main branch (5.4 ± 1.8 to 5.3 ± 1.7 mm³/mm, P = .227), implicating carina shift to account for the change in vessel size (n = 56). The mean side branch FFR was 0.71 ± 0.20 (n = 68) with 43% of lesions being functionally significant. Pre-intervention percent diameter side branch stenosis and the main branch minimum lumen diameter distal to the side branch ostium were independent predictors of functionally significant side branch jailing. In patients with 75% or more stenosis and Thrombolysis in Myocardial Infarction (TIMI) grade 3 flow in the side branch, no difference in post-stent angiographic and IVUS parameters was found between side branch lesions with and

without functional significance. Both plaque shift from the main branch and carina shift contribute to a side branch ostial lesion after main branch stent implantation. Anatomic evaluation does not reliably predict the functional significance of a jailed side branch stenosis.

Saphenous Vein Graft Assessment

Considerations regarding use of FFR in assessing lesions in the saphenous vein graft (SVG) involve two questions. First, is there a difference in FFR when assessing a coronary bypass conduit, and second, what is the fate of the conduit when placed on a vessel for a lesion which is not physiologically significant?

With regard to assessing a lesion in an SVG, there are 3 sources of coronary blood flow to the distal myocardial region: epicardial, conduit flow, and collateral flow. After CABG surgery, the bypass conduit should act in a similar fashion to the native low resistance epicardial vessel supplying the myocardial bed. The assessment of a stenosis in a CABG conduit is must include consideration of the competing flow (and pressure) from (1) the native and conduit vessels; (2) the collateral flow induced from long-standing native coronary occlusion; and (3) the potential for microvascular abnormalities caused by ischemic fibrosis and scarring, preexisting or bypass surgery related MI, or chronic low flow ischemia. In the most uncomplicated situation of an occluded native vessel with minimal distal collateral supply, the theory of FFR should apply just as much to a lesion in an SVG to the right coronary artery feeding a normal myocardial bed as a lesion in the native right coronary. For more complex situations, the FFR of less than 0.08 will reflect the summed responses of the 3 supply sources and yield a net FFR indicating potential ischemia in that region, and vice versa.

With regard to the fate of SVG conduits implanted distal to hemodynamically insignificant lesions, bypass surgeons and cardiologists have recognized that late patency is reduced and native CAD in that vessel can be accelerated.[40] Although most surgical consultations recommend bypassing all lesions with greater than 50% diameter narrowing in patients with multivessel disease, the patency rate of saphenous vein grafts on vessels with hemodynamically nonsignificant lesions has rarely been questioned. Botman and colleagues[41] found that there was a 20% to 25% incidence of graft closure in 450 coronary artery bypass grafts when placed on nonhemodynamically significantly stenosed arteries (preoperative FFR >0.80) at 1-year follow-up (**Fig. 14**). While the precise mechanisms of graft closure remain under study, it is postulated that coronary blood flow favors the

lower resistance path through the native (relatively) nonobstructed arteries rather than vein grafts, with slower or competitive graph flow promoting premature graft closure. In patients requiring CABG for multivessel revascularization, angiographic lesions of uncertain significance would benefit by FFR, providing prognostic information regarding potential of future bypass graft patency. FFR has serious implications for the best long-term CABG outcomes.

Acute Coronary Syndrome

The pathophysiology of the infarct-related artery and bed after MI is complex. Because of the dynamic nature of patients with acute coronary syndrome (ACS), particularly MI, the predictive ability of FFR has some theoretical limitations. In ACS the microvascular bed in the infarct zone may not have uniform, constant, or minimal resistance. The stenosis may also evolve as thrombus and vasoconstriction may abate. FFR measurements are not meaningful when angiographic reperfusion (ie, TIMI 3 flow) not been achieved in the artery. FFR has limited use in the infarct-related artery in the first 24 to 48 hours. However, FFR is has value in lesion assessment in the recovery phase of MI and in the assessment of lesions in the remote noninfarct-related vessels.

To address the utility of measurements days after MI, DeBruyne and colleagues[42] compared SPECT MPI and FFR obtained before and after PCI in 57 MI patients more than 6 days (mean 20 days) prior to evaluation. Patients with positive SPECT before PCI had a significantly lower FFR than patients with negative SPECT (0.52 ± 0.18

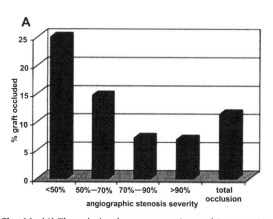
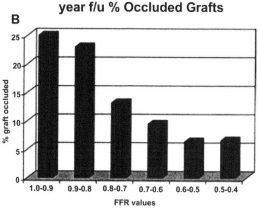

Fig. 14. (*A*) The relation between angiographic stenosis severity and graft failure after angiographic follow-up at 1 year. (*B*) The relation between functional stenosis severity established by fractional flow reserve (FFR) measurements and graft failure at angiographic follow-up after 1 year. (*B, From* Botman CJ, Schonberger J, Koolen S, et al. Does stenosis severity of native vessels influence bypass graft patency? A prospective fractional flow reserve-guided study. Ann Thorac Surg 2007;83:2093–7; with permission.)

vs 0.67 ± 0.16; $P = .0079$), but a significantly higher left ventricular ejection fraction (63% ± 10% vs 52% ± 10%; $P = .0009$) despite a similar percent diameter stenosis (67% ± 13% vs 68% ± 16%; P not significant). The sensitivity and specificity of FFR of less than 0.75 to detect a defect on SPECT were 82% and 87%, respectively. When only truly positive and negative SPECT imaging was considered, the corresponding values were 87% and 100% ($P<.001$). The best FFR cut-off for determining peri-infarct ischemia was 0.78. Of note, a significant inverse correlation was found between left ventricular ejection fraction and FFR ($r = 0.29$, $P = .049$), suggesting a relationship between FFR and the mass of viable myocardium. In a similar study, McClish and colleagues[43] found that FFR values were the same in 43 vessels subtending recent infarct beds 4 days after MI compared with 25 control vessels, matched by lesion length and minimal luminal diameter, in patients without

infarcts (0.67 ± 17 vs 0.68 ± 17, P not significant). Samady and colleagues[44] compared FFR with SPECT and myocardial contrast echo (MCE) in 48 patients 3.7 ± 1.3 days after infarction. To identify true reversibility, follow-up SPECT was performed 11 weeks after PCI. The sensitivity, specificity, and concordance of FFR of 0.75 or less for detecting true reversibility on SPECT were 88%, 93%, and 91% (chi-square $P<.001$), and for detecting reversibility on MCE were 90%, 100%, and 93% (chi-square $P<.001$), respectively (**Fig. 15**). The optimal FFR value for discriminating inducible ischemia on noninvasive imaging was also 0.78, similar to DeBruyne and colleagues.[42]

To predict left ventricular function recovery after ST-segment elevation myocardial infarction (STEMI), Fearon and colleagues[24] found that patients with preserved IMR after primary angioplasty may have greater recovery of regional ventricular function after primary angioplasty for

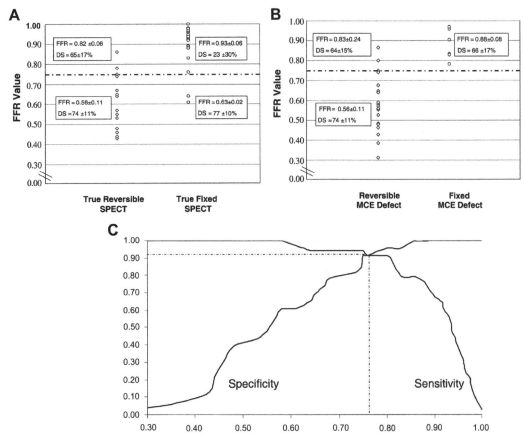

Fig. 15. (*A*) Concordance between FFR and SPECT (DP-stress paired with rest imaging). (*B*) Concordance between FFR and MCE. (*C*) Sensitivity and specificity curves of fractional flow reserve for detecting reversibility of combined noninvasive testing in ACS patients. (*C, From* Samady H, Lepper W, Powers ER, et al. Fractional flow reserve of infarct-related arteries identifies reversible defects on noninvasive myocardial perfusion imaging early after myocardial infarction. J Am Coll Cardiol 2006;47:2187–93; with permission.)

STEMI. In addition to providing prognostic information in this important patient subset, IMR may potentially be used in selecting patients with relatively preserved postinfarct microvasculature that might most benefit from regional delivery of regenerative cell therapies.

For patients with non-STEMI, Leesar and colleagues[45] randomized 70 patients with recent unstable angina or non-STEMI with intermediate single-vessel stenosis to one of two strategies: angiography followed by SPECT the next day or FFR-guided revascularization at the time of angiography. Compared with the SPECT strategy, the FFR-guided approach had a reduced hospital duration (11 ± 2 hours vs 49 ± 5 hours, $P<.001$) and cost ($1329 ± $44 vs $2113 ± $120, $P<.05$), with no increase in procedure time, radiation exposure time, or clinical event rates at 1-year follow-up. Similarly, Potvin and colleagues[46]

evaluated 201 consecutive patients (62% with unstable angina or MI), in whom revascularization was guided by FFR. At 11 ± 6 months of follow-up, cardiac events occurred in 20 patients (10%), and no significant differences were observed between patients with unstable angina or MI and those with stable angina (9% vs 13%, $P = .44$). Finally, Fischer and colleagues[47] found similar MACE rates at 12 months in patients with (n = 35) and without (n = 85) ACS in whom revascularization was guided by FFR (15% vs 9%, P not significant).

Serial (Multiple) Lesions in a Single Vessel

When more than one discrete stenosis is present in the same vessel, the hyperemic flow and pressure gradient through the first one will be attenuated by the presence of the second one, and

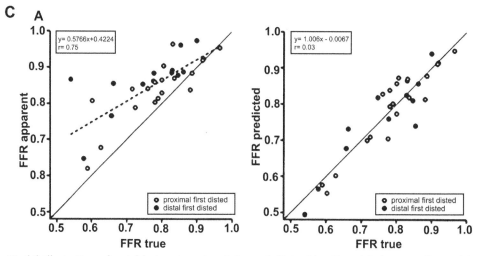

Fig. 16. (*A*) Illustration of serial lesions in epicardial vessel. Note: Max Flow (*a*) changes after resistance (*b*) is reduced. (*B*) Calculation of FFR predicted for serial lesion individually. (*C*) Comparison of predicted and measured FFR in serial lesions. (*C, From* Pijls NH, De Bruyne B, Bech GJ, et al. Coronary pressure measurement to assess the hemodynamic significance of serial stenoses within one coronary artery: validation in humans. Circulation 2000;102:2371–77; with permission.)

A

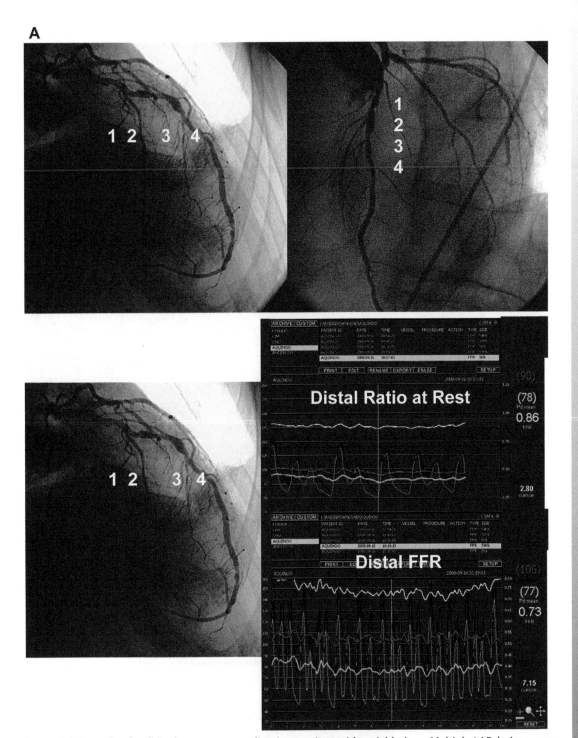

Fig. 17. (*A*) Example of pull-back pressure recording in a patient with serial lesions. Multiple LAD lesions were seen on angiography in a patient with positive stress test for anterior ischemia. Upper and lower left panels are cine angiographic frames showing the 4 lesions. (*Lower right*) the translesional pressure ratio (Pd/Pa) at rest across all lesions was 0.86 but FFR, which summed the 4 lesions, was 0.73.

B

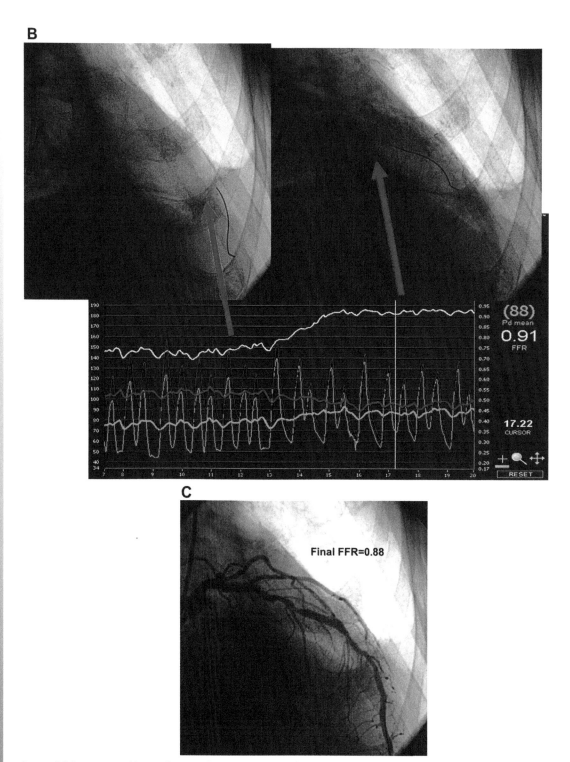

Fig. 17. (*B*) (*Upper panels*) Cine frames of wire positions before and after pull-back of pressure wire. Pressure pull-back shown in lower panel identified step-up of gradient at lesion 3 only. (*C*) Cine frame of LAD after stenting of lesion 3 with a final FFR across all lesions of 0.88.

vice versa (**Fig. 16**). One stenosis will mask the true effect on its serial counterpart by limiting the achievable maximum hyperemia. This fluid dynamic interaction between two serial stenoses depends on the sequence, severity, and distance between the lesions as well as the flow rate. When the distance between two lesions is greater than 6 times the vessel diameter, the stenoses generally behave independently and the overall pressure gradient is the sum of the individual pressure losses at any given flow rate.[48]

When addressing two stenoses in series, equations have been derived to predict the FFR (FFR_{pred}) of each stenosis separately (ie, as if the other one were removed) using arterial pressure (P_a), pressure between the two stenoses (P_m), distal coronary pressure (P_d), and coronary occlusive pressure (P_w). FFR_{app} (ratio of the pressure just distal to that just proximal to each stenosis) and FFR_{true} (ratio of the pressures distal and proximal to each stenosis but after removal of the other one) have been compared in instrumented dogs[48] and in patients.[49] FFR_{true} was more overestimated by FFR_{app} than by FFR_{pred}. It was clearly demonstrated that the interaction between two stenoses is such that the FFR of each lesion separately cannot be calculated by the equation for isolated stenoses applied to each separately, but can be predicted by more complete equations taking into account P_a, P_m, P_d, and P_w.

Although calculation of the exact FFR of each lesion separately is possible, it remains academic. In clinical practice, the use of the pressure pullback recording is particularly well suited to identify the several regions of a vessel with large pressure gradients that may benefit by treatment. The one stenosis with the largest gradient can be treated first, and the FFR can be remeasured for the remaining stenoses to determine the need for further treatment (**Fig. 17**).

Diffuse Coronary Disease

A diffusely diseased atherosclerotic coronary artery can be viewed as a series of branching units diverting and gradually distributing flow along the longitudinally narrowing conduit length. The perfusion pressure gradually diminishes along the artery. In this artery, CFR is reduced but is unassociated with a focal stenotic pressure loss. Thus mechanical therapy directed at a presumed "culprit" plaque to reverse such abnormal physiology would be ineffective in restoring normal coronary perfusion. Using FFR_{myo} during continuous pressure wire pull-back from a distal to proximal location, the impact of a specific area of angiographic narrowing can be examined and

the presence of diffuse atherosclerosis can be documented.[50] Diffuse atherosclerosis, rather than a focal narrowing, is characterized by a continuous and gradual pressure recovery without localized abrupt increase in pressure related to an isolated region. De Bruyne and colleagues[51] have demonstrated the influence of diffuse atherosclerosis that often remains invisible at angiography. FFR_{myo} measurements were obtained from 37 arteries in 10 individuals without atherosclerosis (group I) and from 106 nonstenotic arteries in 62 patients with angiographic stenoses in another coronary artery (group II). In group I, the pressure gradient between aorta and distal coronary artery was minimal at rest (1 ± 1 mm Hg) and during maximal hyperemia (3 ± 3 mm Hg). Corresponding values were significantly larger in group II (5 ± 4 mm Hg and 10 ± 8 mm Hg, respectively; both $P<.001$). The FFR_{myo} was near unity (0.97 ± 0.02; range, 0.92–1) in group I, indicating no resistance to flow in truly normal coronary arteries, but it was significantly lower (0.89 ± 0.08; range, 0.69–1) in group II, indicating a higher resistance to flow (**Fig 18**). This resistance to flow contributes to myocardial ischemia and has consequences for decision making during PCI.

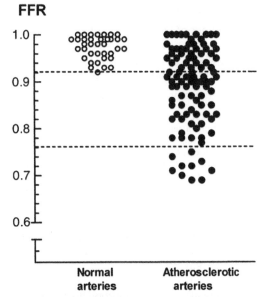

Fig. 18. Graphs of individual values of FFR in normal arteries and in atherosclerotic coronary arteries without focal stenosis on arteriogram. The upper dashed line indicates the lowest value of FFR in normal coronary arteries. The lower dashed line indicates the 0.75 threshold level. (*Reproduced from* De Bruyne B, Hersbach F, Pijls NH, et al. Abnormal epicardial coronary resistance in patients with diffuse atherosclerosis but "normal" coronary angiography. Circulation 2001;104:2401–6; with permission.)

Box 3
Current role of physiologic measurements in the cath lab

PCI Guideline Recommended Uses

1. Assessment of the effects of intermediate coronary stenoses (30%–70% luminal narrowing) in patients with anginal symptoms. Coronary pressure or Doppler velocimetry may also be useful as an alternative to performing noninvasive functional testing (eg, when the functional study is absent or ambiguous) to determine whether an intervention is warranted (Class IIa, *Level of Evidence: B*)
2. Assessing the success of PCI in restoring flow reserve and to predict the risk of restenosis (Class IIb, *Level of Evidence: C*)
3. Evaluating patients with anginal symptoms without an apparent angiographic culprit lesion (Class IIb, *Level of Evidence: C*)
4. Routine assessment of the severity of angiographic disease in patients with a positive, unequivocal noninvasive functional study is not recommended (Class III, *Level of Evidence: C*)

Applications of FFR Under Study[a]:

1. Determination of one or more culprit stenoses (either serially or in separate vessels) in patients with multivessel disease
2. Evaluation of ostial or distal left main and ostial right lesions, especially when these regions cannot be well visualized by angiography
3. Guidance of treatment of serial stenoses in a coronary artery
4. Determination of significance of focal treatable region in vessel with diffuse CAD
5. Determination of prognosis after stent deployment
6. Assessment of stenosis in patients with previous (nonacute, >6 days) MI
7. Assessment of lesions in patients with treated unstable angina pectoris
8. Assessment of the collateral circulation

Applications of Coronary Doppler Flow Under Study[a]

1. Assessment of microcirculation
2. Endothelial function testing
3. Myocardial viability in acute MI

Applications of Combined Coronary Pressure and Doppler Flow Velocity Under Study[a]

1. Assessment of intermediate stenosis
2. Assessment of the microcirculation
3. Identification of lesion compliance (change of pressure-velocity relationship)

[a] Not yet recommended by PCI Guidelines.

From Smith SC Jr, Feldman TE, Hirshfeld JW Jr, et al. ACC/AHA/SCAI 2005 guideline update for percutaneous coronary intervention: a report of the American College of Cardiology/American Heart Association Task Force on Practice Guidelines (ACC/AHA/SCAI Writing Committee to Update the 2001 Guidelines for Percutaneous Coronary Intervention). American College of Cardiology Foundation and the American Heart Association, Inc. Cardiology Web Site. Available at: http://www.acc.org/clinical/guidelines/percutaneous/update/index.pdf. Accessed January 13, 2011; with permission.

The pressure pull-back recording at maximum hyperemia will provide the necessary information to decide if and where stent implantation may be useful (see **Fig. 17**). The location of a focal pressure drop superimposed on the diffuse disease can be identified as an appropriate location for treatment.

FFR AND THE COLLATERAL CIRCULATION

The collateral circulation can be described by intracoronary pressure and flow relationships. Ipsilateral collateral flow and contralateral arterial responses have been described in numerous studies using both pressure and flow to provide new information regarding mechanisms, function, and clinical significance of collateral flow in patients.[52,53] To improve the conventional angiographic assessment of collateral supply, FFR of the collateral flow employs the use of coronary occlusion wedge pressure. FFR collateral greater than 0.25–0.30 is associated with good collateralization and often nonischemic evaluations of provocable outpatient ischemia.[54]

SUMMARY

FFR is considered as one of the standards for functional assessment of CAD, acting as a single-vessel stress test within the cardiac cath lab environment.

Although the cost of the physiologic information translates into an operational expense for the catheterization laboratory, the data identify significant overall savings to the health care system and a substantial clinical benefit to the patient.

FFR use in the cath lab has steadily grown over the past decade and, given the strong case for favorable outcomes in a variety of common and complex anatomic subset, FFR has evident clinical value for decision making in the laboratory. **Box 3** lists the current role of physiology for decision making in the cath lab.[11] FFR technology has overcome the hurdles of cumbersome setup time and concerns regarding accurate hemodynamics. Physiologic data acquired during the angiographic procedure can facilitate timely, as well as clinically and economically sound decision making to direct revascularization options for best patient outcomes.

REFERENCES

1. Pijls NH, DeBruyne B, Peels K, et al. Measurement of fractional flow reserve to assess the functional severity of coronary-artery stenoses. N Engl J Med 1996;334:1703–8.

2. Pijls NH, Van Gelder B, Van der Voort P, et al. Fractional flow reserve: a useful index to evaluate the influence of an epicardial coronary stenosis on myocardial blood flow. Circulation 1995;92:318–9.

3. Bech GJ, DeBruyne B, Pijls NH, et al. Fractional flow reserve to determine the appropriateness of angioplasty in moderate coronary stenosis: a randomized trial. Circulation 2001;103(24):2928–34.

4. Pijls NH, Van Schaardenburgh P, Manoharan G, et al. Percutaneous coronary intervention of functionally non-significant stenoses: 5-year follow-up of the DEFER study. J Am Coll Cardiol 2007;49: 2105–11.

5. Koo BK, Kang HJ, Youn TJ, et al. Physiologic assessment of jailed side branch lesions using fractional flow reserve. J Am Coll Cardiol 2005;46(4):633–7.

6. Ziaee A, Parham WA, Herrmann SC, et al. Lack of relation between imaging and physiology in ostial coronary artery narrowings. Am J Cardiol 2004; 93(11):1404–7 A9.

7. Pijls NH, Fearon WF, Tonino PA, et al. Fractional flow reserve versus angiography for guiding percutaneous coronary intervention in patients with multivessel coronary artery disease: 2-year follow-up of the FAME (Fractional Flow Reserve Versus Angiography for Multivessel Evaluation) study. J Am Coll Cardiol 2010;56:177–84.

8. Berger A, Botman KJ, MacCarthy PA, et al. Long-term clinical outcome after fractional flow reserve-guided percutaneous coronary intervention in patients with multivessel disease. J Am Coll Cardiol 2005;46:438–42.

9. Bech GJ, Droste H, Pijls NH, et al. Value of fractional flow reserve in making decisions about bypass surgery for equivocal left main coronary artery disease. Heart 2001;86(5):547–52.

10. Hamilos M, Muller O, Cuisset T, et al. Long-term clinical outcome after fractional flow reserve–guided treatment in patients with angiographically equivocal left main coronary artery stenosis. Circulation 2009;120:1505–12.

11. Kern MJ, Lerman A, Bech JW, et al. Physiological assessment of coronary artery disease in the cardiac catheterization laboratory: a scientific statement from the American Heart Association Committee on Diagnostic and Interventional Cardiac Catheterization. Circulation 2006;114(12):1321–41.

12. Topol EJ, Nissen SE. Our preoccupation with coronary luminology. The dissociation between clinical and angiographic findings in ischemic heart disease. Circulation 1995;92:2333–42.

13. Meijboom WB, Van Mieghem CA, van Pelt N, et al. Comprehensive assessment of coronary artery stenoses: computed tomography coronary angiography versus conventional coronary angiography and correlation with fractional flow reserve in patients with stable angina. J Am Coll Cardiol 2008;52(8):636–43.

14. Spaan JA, Piek JJ, Hoofman JI, et al. Physiological basis of clinically used coronary hemodynamic indices. Circulation 2006;113:446–55.

15. Pijls NH, DeBruyne B. Coronary pressure. Dordrecht (The Netherlands): Kluwer Academic Publishers; 1998.

16. Pijls NHJ, Kern MJ, Yock PG, et al. Practice and potential pitfalls of coronary pressure measurement. Catheter Cardiovasc Interv 2000;49:1–16.

17. DeBruyne B, Bartunek J, Sys SU, et al. Relation between myocardial fractional flow reserve calculated from coronary pressure measurements and exercise-induced myocardial ischemia. Circulation 1995;92:39–46.

18. McGeoch RJ, Oldroyd KG. Pharmacological options for inducing maximal hyperaemia during studies of coronary physiology. Catheter Cardiovasc Interv 2008;71:198–204.

19. Jeremias A, Whitbourn RJ, Filardo SD, et al. Adequacy of intracoronary versus intravenous adenosine-induced maximal coronary hyperemia for fractional flow reserve measurements. Am Heart J 2000;140(4):651–7.

20. Ntalianis A, Trana C, Muller O, et al. Effective radiation dose, time, and contrast medium to measure fractional flow reserve. JACC Cardiovasc Interv 2010;3:821–7.

21. Kern MJ, Samady H. Current concepts of integrated coronary physiology in the cath lab. J Am Coll Cardiol 2010;55:173–85.

22. Christou MA, Siontis GC, Katritsis DG, et al. Meta-analysis of fractional flow reserve versus quantitative coronary angiography and noninvasive imaging for evaluation of myocardial ischemia. Am J Cardiol 2007;99(4):450–6.

23. Meuwissen M, Chamuleau SAJ, Siebes M, et al. The prognostic value of combined intracoronary pressure and blood flow velocity measurements after deferral of percutaneous coronary intervention. Catheter Cardiovasc Interv 2008;71:291–7.

24. Fearon WF, Shah M, Ng M, et al. Predictive value of the index of microcirculatory resistance in patients with ST-segment elevation myocardial infarction. J Am Coll Cardiol 2008;51:560–5.

25. Siebes M, Verhoeff BJ, Meuwissen M, et al. Single-wire pressure and flow velocity measurement to quantify coronary stenosis hemodynamics and effects of percutaneous interventions. Circulation 2004;109:756–62.

26. Watkins S, Chir B, McGeoch R, et al. Validation of magnetic resonance myocardial perfusion imaging with fractional flow reserve for the detection of significant coronary heart disease. Circulation 2009;120: 2207–13.

27. Melikian N, De Bondt P, Tonino P, et al. Fractional flow reserve and myocardial perfusion imaging in patients with angiographic multivessel coronary artery disease. JACC Cardiovasc Interv 2010;3: 307–14.

28. Magni V, Chieffo A, Colombo A. Evaluation of intermediate coronary stenosis with intravascular ultrasound and fractional flow reserve: its use and abuse. Catheter Cardiovasc Interv 2009;73:441–8.

29. Takagi A, Tsurumi Y, Ishii Y, et al. Clinical potential of intravascular ultrasound for physiological assessment of coronary stenosis. Relationship between quantitative ultrasound tomography and pressure-derived fractional flow reserve. Circulation 1999; 100:250–5.

30. Iqbal MB, Shah N, Khan M, et al. Reduction in myocardial perfusion territory and its effect on the physiological severity of a coronary stenosis. Circ Cardiovasc Interv Feb 2010;3:89–90.

31. Abizaid A, Mintz G, Mehran R, et al. Long-term follow-up after percutaneous transluminal coronary angioplasty was not performed based on intravascular ultrasound findings: importance of lumen dimensions. Circulation 1999;100:256–61.

32. Takayama T, Hodgson JM. Prediction of the physiologic severity of coronary lesions using 3-D IVUS: validation by direct coronary pressure measurements. Catheter Cardiovasc Interv 2001;53:48–55.

33. Nam C-W, Yoon H-J, Cho Y-K, et al. Outcomes of percutaneous coronary intervention in intermediate coronary artery disease: fractional flow reserve–guided versus intravascular ultrasound–guided. JACC Cardiovasc Interv 2010;3:812–7.

34. Tonino PAL, Fearon WF, De Bruyne B, et al. Angiographic versus functional severity of coronary artery stenoses in the FAME study, fractional flow reserve versus angiography in multivessel evaluation. J Am Coll Cardiol 2010;55:2816–21.

35. Sant'Anna FM, Silva EE, Batista LA, et al. Influence of routine assessment of fractional flow reserve on decision making during coronary interventions. Am J Cardiol 2007;99:504–8.

36. Tonino PA, DeBruyne B, Pijls NH, et al. Fractional flow reserve versus angiography for guiding percutaneous coronary intervention. N Engl J Med 2009; 360(3):213–24.

37. Samady H, McDaniel M, Veledar E, et al. Baseline fractional flow reserve and stent diameter predict optimal post-stent fractional flow reserve and major adverse cardiac events after bare-metal stent deployment. JACC Cardiovasc Interv 2009;2: 357–63.

38. Koo BK, Park KW, Kang HJ, et al. Physiological evaluation of the provisional side-branch intervention strategy for bifurcation lesions using fractional flow reserve. Eur Heart J 2008;29(6):726–32.

39. Koo BK, Waseda K, Kang HJ, et al. Anatomic and functional evaluation of bifurcation lesions undergoing percutaneous coronary intervention. Circ Cardiovasc Interv 2010;3:113–9.

40. Berger A, MacCarthy PA, Vanermen H, et al. Occlusion of internal mammary grafts: a review of the potential causative factors. Acta Chir Belg 2004; 104(6):630–4.

41. Botman CJ, Schonberger J, Koolen S, et al. Does stenosis severity of native vessels influence bypass graft patency? a prospective fractional flow reserve-guided study. Ann Thorac Surg 2007;83:2093–7.

42. DeBruyne B, Pijls NHJ, Bartunek J, et al. Fractional flow reserve in patients with prior myocardial infarction. Circulation 2001;104:157–62.

43. McClish JC, Ragosta M, Powers ER, et al. Recent myocardial infarction does not limit the utility of fractional flow reserve for the physiologic assessment of lesion severity. Am J Cardiol 2004;93(9):1102–6.

44. Samady H, Lepper W, Powers ER, et al. Fractional flow reserve of infarct-related arteries identifies reversible defects on noninvasive myocardial perfusion imaging early after myocardial infarction. J Am Coll Cardiol 2006;47:2187–93.

45. Leesar MA, Abdul-Baki T, Akkus NI, et al. Use of fractional flow reserve versus stress perfusion scintigraphy after unstable angina. Effect on duration of hospitalization, cost, procedural characteristics, and clinical outcome. J Am Coll Cardiol 2003;41: 1115–21.

46. Potvin JM, Rodés-Cabau J, Bertrand OF, et al. Usefulness of fractional flow reserve measurements to defer revascularization in patients with stable or unstable angina pectoris, non-ST-elevation and

ST-elevation acute myocardial infarction, or atypical chest pain. Am J Cardiol 2006;98:289–97.

47. Fischer JJ, Wang XQ, Samady H, et al. Outcome of patients with acute coronary syndromes and moderate lesions undergoing deferral of revascularization based on fractional flow reserve assessment. Catheter Cardiovasc Interv 2006;68:544–8.

48. De Bruyne B, Pijls NH, Heyndrickx GR, et al. Pressure-derived fractional flow reserve to assess serial epicardial stenoses: theoretical basis and animal validation. Circulation 2000;101:1840–7.

49. Pijls NH, De Bruyne B, Bech GJ, et al. Coronary pressure measurement to assess the hemodynamic significance of serial stenoses within one coronary artery: validation in humans. Circulation 2000;102:2371–7.

50. Pijls NH, Bech GJ, el Gamal MI, et al. Quantification of recruitable coronary collateral blood flow in conscious humans and its potential to predict future ischemic events. J Am Coll Cardiol 1995;25:1522–8.

51. DeBruyne B, Hersbach F, Pijls NH, et al. Abnormal epicardial coronary resistance in patients with diffuse atherosclerosis but normal coronary angiography. Circulation 2001;104:2401–6.

52. Piek JJ, van Liebergen RA, Koch KT, et al. Clinical, angiographic and hemodynamic predictors of recruitable collateral flow assessed during balloon angioplasty coronary occlusion. J Am Coll Cardiol 1997;29:275–82.

53. Pohl T, Seiler C, Billinger M, et al. Frequency distribution of collateral flow and factors influencing collateral channel development: functional collateral channel measurement in 450 patients with coronary artery disease. J Am Coll Cardiol 2001;38:1872–8.

54. Werner GS, Ferrari M, Betge S, et al. Collateral function in chronic total coronary occlusions is related to regional myocardial function and duration of occlusion. Circulation 2001;104:2784–90.

55. Bartunek J, Van Schuerbeeck E, DeBruyne B. Comparison of exercise electrocardiography and Dobutamine echocardiography with invasively assessed myocardial fractional flow reserve in evaluation of severity of coronary arterial narrowing. Am J Cardiol 1997;79:478–81.

56. Abe M, Tomiyama H, Yoshida H, et al. Diastolic fractional flow reserve to assess the functional severity of moderate coronary artery stenoses: comparison with fractional flow reserve and coronary flow velocity reserve. Circulation 2000;102:2365–70.

57. Chamuleau SA, Meuwissen M, van Eck-Smit BL, et al. Fractional flow reserve, absolute and relative coronary blood flow velocity reserve in relation to the results of technetium-99m sestamibi single-photon emission computed tomography in patients with two vessel coronary artery disease. J Am Coll Cardiol 2001;37:1316–22.

58. Caymaz O, Fak AS, Tezcan H, et al. Correlation of myocardial fraction flow reserve with thallium-201 SPECT imaging in intermediate-severity coronary artery lesions. J Invasive Cardiol 2000;12:345–50 [published comment in J Invasive Cardiol 2000;12:351–3].

59. Jimenez-Navarro M, Alonso-Briales JH, Hernandez Garcia MJ, et al. Measurement of fractional flow reserve to assess moderately severe coronary lesions: correlation with Dobutamine stress echocardiography. J Interv Cardiol 2001;14:499–504.

60. Usui Y, Chikamori T, Yanagisawa H, et al. Reliability of pressure-derived myocardial fractional flow reserve in assessing coronary artery stenosis in patients with previous myocardial infarction. Am J Cardiol 2003;92:699–702.

61. Yanagisawa H, Chikamori T, Tanaka N, et al. Correlation between thallium-201 myocardial perfusion defects and the functional severity of coronary artery stenosis as assessed by pressure-derived myocardial fractional flow reserve. Circ J 2002;66:1105–9.

62. Courtis J, Rodés-Cabau J, Larose E, et al. Usefulness of coronary fractional flow reserve measurements in guiding clinical decisions in intermediate or equivocal left main coronary stenoses. Am J Cardiol 2009;103(76):943–9.

63. Lindstaedt M, Yazar A, Germing A, et al. Clinical outcome in patients with intermediate or equivocal left main coronary artery disease after deferral of surgical revascularization on the basis of fractional flow reserve measurements. Am Heart J 2006;152(1):156, e1–9

64. Suemaru S, Iwasaki K, Yamamoto K, et al. Coronary pressure measurement to determine treatment strategy for equivocal left main coronary artery lesions. Heart Vessels 2005;20:271–7.

65. Legutko J, Dudek D, Rzeszutko L, et al. Fractional flow reserve assessment to determine the indications for myocardial revascularization in patients with borderline stenosis of the left main coronary artery. Kardiol Pol 2005;63:499–509.

66. Jimenez-Navarro M, Hernandez-Garcia JM, Alonso-Briales JH, et al. Should we treat patients with moderately severe stenosis of the left main coronary artery and negative FFR results? J Invas Cardiol 2004;16:398–400.

Invasive Hemodynamic Assessment in Heart Failure

Barry A. Borlaug, MD[a],*, David A. Kass, MD[b]

KEYWORDS

- Hemodynamics • Heart failure • Systole • Diastole
- Ventricular-arterial interaction • Cardiovascular function

The concept of hemodynamics was born in 1628 with Harvey's description of the circulation, but its growth was limited for centuries by the inability to measure pressure and flow accurately. The work of Starling, Wiggers, and other hemodynamic physiologists in the first part of the twentieth century, along with introduction of cardiac catheterization by Cournand and Richards in the 1940s ushered in the golden era of hemodynamics. From the late 1970s to early 1990s, there was an explosion of clinical and basic research as new methods were developed to quantify ventricular systolic and diastolic properties more definitively. Enthusiasm for such characterization subsequently waned, however, as therapies directly targeting hemodynamic derangements, such as inotropes, were found to hasten mortality. This change coincided with a paradigm shift in the way heart failure was conceptualized, from a disease of abnormal hemodynamics to one of neurohormonal derangements, abnormal cell signaling, and maladaptive remodeling. As such, many "gold-standard" methods for characterizing load, contractility, diastole, and, ventricular-arterial interaction were not adopted into clinical practice. A working understanding of each element remains paramount to interpret properly the hemodynamic changes in patients who have acute and chronic heart failure, however.

Routine cardiac catheterization provides data on left heart, right heart, systemic and pulmonary arterial pressures, vascular resistances, cardiac output, and ejection fraction. These data are often then applied as markers of cardiac preload, afterload, and global function, although each of these parameters reflects more complex interactions between the heart and its internal and external loads. This article reviews more specific, gold standard assessments of ventricular and arterial properties and how these relate to the parameters reported and used in practice, and then discusses the re-emerging importance of invasive hemodynamics in the assessment and management of heart failure.

CARDIAC CONTRACTILITY: LOOKING BEYOND THE EJECTION FRACTION

The most universally accepted index of contractility used in practice, the EF, unfortunately is also one of the least specific.[1] As with any parameter measuring the extent of muscle shortening or thickening, it is highly sensitive to afterload and really is an expression of ventricular–arterial coupling rather than of contractility alone. EF also is affected by heart size, because its denominator is end-diastolic volume (EDV), leading many to propose that EF is more a parameter of remodeling than of contractility. EF commonly is used to classify different "forms" of heart failure (low vs preserved EF).[2] This approach is appealing, given its binary nature and ease of application in practice, but the realities of how a patient develops signs and symptoms of heart failure are far more complex,[3] and in this regard EF serves as a somewhat arbitrary marker.

More specific measures of contractility have been developed but because of their complexity

This article originally appeared in *Heart Failure Clinics*, volume 5, number 2.

[a] Mayo Clinic and Foundation, Rochester, MN, USA

[b] Johns Hopkins Medical Institutions, Baltimore, MD, USA

* Corresponding author. Division of Cardiovascular Diseases, Department of Medicine, Mayo Clinic and Foundation, Gonda 5-455, 200 First Street SW, Rochester, MN 55905.

E-mail address: borlaug.barry@mayo.edu

remain used principally in research. The maximal rate of pressure rise during isovolumic contraction (dP/dt_{max}) can be assessed using a high-fidelity micromanometer and is used widely as a measure of contractility. dP/dt_{max}, however, is dependent on cardiac filling (ie, is preload dependent) and heart rate, and it may not always reflect contractile function that develops after cardiac ejection is initiated.[4] In patients who have cardiac dyssynchrony, the lack of coordinated contraction in early-systole reduces dP/dt_{max} because the force developed by the early activated wall is dissipated by stretching of the still relaxed opposite wall.[5] dP/dt_{max} is quite sensitive to this phenomenon (**Fig. 1**), but in this case it reflects chamber mechanics rather than intrinsic muscle function.

An ideal parameter of contractility would assess inotropic state independently of preload, afterload, heart rate, and remodeling.[1] This assessment still

remains somewhat elusive, but parameters derived from relations between cardiac pressure and volume have come the closest to achieving it. As shown in **Fig. 1**B, a series of variably loaded pressure–volume (PV) loops can be obtained to assess systolic, diastolic, coupling, and energetic properties. Stroke work, dP/dt_{max}, maximal ventricular power, elastance, efficiency, and other parameters are assessed, and by examining these variables over a range of preload volumes, one can derive more load-independent, cardiac-specific measures.[6]

The relationship between end-systolic pressure and volume from a variety of variably loaded cardiac contractions yields the end-systolic pressure volume relationship (ESPVR),[7] its slope being the end-systolic elastance (Ees) (see **Fig. 1**B). The Ees conveys information about both contractile function and myocardial

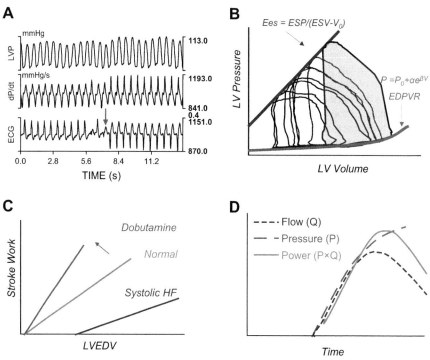

Fig. 1. (*A*) Time plot of left ventricular pressure (LVP), first derivative of pressure (dP/dt), and EKG in a patient who has heart failure with left bundle-type conduction delay. At the arrow, the patient received bi-ventricular stimulation resulting in an abrupt rise in dP/dt_{max}. (*B*) PV loops obtained at baseline and during transient caval occlusion (decreasing LV volumes—loops moving right to left). The slope of the EDSPV derived from multibeat analysis defines ventricular Ees, a load-independent measure of contractility. By measuring diastolic pressure and volume during diastasis at variably loaded beats, the end-diastolic PV relationship (EDPVR) is obtained. The shaded area subtended by the baseline loop represents the stroke work performed by the ventricle. ESP, end-systolic pressure; ESV, end-systolic volume; V_0, volume axis intercept of ESPVR. (*C*) The slope of the relation between systolic chamber performance (stroke work) and preload (left ventricle end-diastolic volume, LVEDV) determines the preload recruitable stroke work. This relationship shifts up and to the left, as indicated by the arrow, with an increase in contractility, as with dobutamine, or down and to the right with systolic heart failure (HF). (*D*) LV power (P × Q, *solid line*) is determined by the product of simultaneously measured pressure (P, *dashed line*) and flow (Q, *dotted line*). When indexed to preload, this calculation produces another load-independent measure of LV chamber contractility.

constitutive properties; that is, it is a measure of chamber stiffness. It can be related easily to arterial vascular load to assess ventricular–arterial interaction[8] and provides important information about how a patient's blood pressure and flow will respond to loading changes.[9] Although traditionally Ees was assessed from multiple cardiac cycles requiring simultaneous measurement of cardiac pressure and volume (or flow), algorithms have been generated and tested to derive these parameters noninvasively from single steady-state data.[10–12] These parameters have been used to characterize systolic properties in various forms of heart failure and in larger populations.[6,13,14] The diastolic correlate of Ees is the end-diastolic elastance, the lower PV boundary that is parameterized most often by a mono-exponential stiffness coefficient. Both the Ees and diastolic curve fits are dependent on chamber size and remodeling.

Several other parameters commonly are derived for indexing systolic function. The relationship between stroke work and preload, measured from multiple beats under different loading generates a "Sarnoff curve," and its slope, often termed "preload recruitable stroke work" (PRSW) provides a contractile index (see **Fig. 1**C).[15] Maximal ventricular power (PWR$_{max}$) is the peak instantaneous product of ventricular outflow and pressure and also is quite preload dependent (see **Fig. 1**D).

Regression over a range of preloads yields a more specific index, however, and because the intercept of this relation often is near zero for normal-sized ventricles, the ratio of PWR$_{max}$/EDV can be used. In failing ventricles, normalization to EDV^2 seems to reduce load dependence better.[16,17]

DIASTOLE—MORE THAN END-DIASTOLIC PRESSURE

Diastolic function is determined from active and passive processes, and both contribute to relaxation and chamber filling.[3] Left heart filling pressures, either pulmonary artery occlusion (wedge pressure) or left ventricle (LV) end-diastolic pressure (EDP), are central to standard cardiac catheterization, and their elevation is taken to reflect abnormal loading and/or abnormal chamber compliance. One cannot determine whether the elevation reflects abnormal loading or abnormal chamber compliance from the pressure parameter alone, but diastolic function also is assessed by a variety of noninvasive methods to characterize it better.

Aortic valve closure marks the onset of ventricular diastole, where relaxation is quantified invasively by the rate of pressure decay, typically expressed by a time constant (τ) that is estimated using a number of mathematical fits (**Fig. 2**).[18]

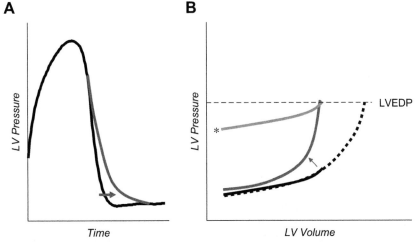

Fig. 2. (*A*) The kinetics of LV pressure decay during isovolumic relaxation (the time between aortic valve closure and mitral opening) can be modeled by various equations to derive the time constant, τ. The curve indicated by the arrow shows prolonged relaxation, often seen with heart failure, aging, and hypertension. (*B*) Groups of DPVR. The solid black line shows the curve in a normal person. The curve that shifts up and to the left (*arrow*) indicates the effects of increased passive chamber stiffness. Filling pressures (LVEDP) may be elevated because of the increased passive chamber stiffness, but similar elevations also can be seen in the absence of increased stiffness, as when there is with increased extrinsic restraint (line indicated by the *asterisk*). Note that the shape (stiffness) of the DPVR with enhanced restraint is similar to that in the normal patient. Finally, EDP may be elevated simply because of the overfilling of a structurally normal ventricle (*dotted black line*). There is evidence to support each of these possible contributors to elevated EDP in HFpEF.

Even this seemingly straightforward assessment has technical pitfalls. These model fits—usually mono-exponential decays (ie, $P = P_\infty + P_o e^{-t/\tau}$, or the same equation without P_∞)—may or may not describe adequately the actual fall of pressure. When used in a setting where they do not fit properly, such as in dilated heart failure, they can lead to erroneous conclusions.[18] An alternative model based on a modified logistic equation, $P = P_A/(1 + e^{t/\tau}) + P_B$,[19] fits such failure data better than the exponential. Chung and Kovacs[20] recently explored both model fits in contrast to a more physics-based approach, showing that relaxation is best described using both resistive and elastic elements. This intriguing approach deserves further attention in clinical studies.

Delayed relaxation is common. It frequently accompanies normal aging,[21] but it becomes even more prominent in cardiac failure and with hypertrophy. It has multiple determinants starting with dissociation of the cross-bridge, calcium-handling, and elasticity-restoring forces resulting from the recoil of compressed macromolecules such as titin.[3] The extent to which delayed relaxation alters mean and late-diastolic pressures remains controversial,[22] because diastole generally is long enough that even delayed relaxation is completed before late-diastolic filling occurs. It clearly can affect early filling and pressures, particularly at faster heart rates. Analysis requires invasive high-fidelity micromanometer recordings, although it may be approximated by the time between aortic valve closure and mitral valve opening or inferred from mitral Doppler flow patterns.[23]

Similar to isovolumic relaxation, passive diastolic chamber stiffness rarely is measured directly in standard clinical practice. As noted, the LV diastolic pressure–volume relationship (DPVR; see **Fig. 1B**) is curvilinear; thus compliance most often is expressed by a mono-exponential stiffness coefficient.[24] Linear approximations have been used, but one must be careful to compare these approximations within similar loading ranges. The DPVR most often is estimated from a single heartbeat, although this estimation combines features that reflect early relaxation and resistive (viscous) properties and extra-chamber (eg, pericardial) loading. A more accurate approach is to assess multiple PV loops over a loading range (varying preload) and to connect points at late-diastole from these cycles (see **Fig. 1B**). The apparent chamber stiffness derived from single versus multiple loops can vary substantially, as shown particularly in patients who have genetic hypertrophic cardiomyopathy; in these patients the use of a single loop markedly underestimated LV stiffness.[25]

LVEDP may be increased because chamber is stiffer or is subject to higher preload or because the entire DPVR is shifted upwards (see **Fig. 2B**).[3] All three variables play a role in heart failure with a reduced EF. The first and last seem to contribute mostly to heart failure with a preserved EF (HFpEF),[14,26,27] and although some have found increased LV filling volumes as well,[28] this phenomenon has not been seen by others.[14,29] Approximately 40% of a measured intracavitary LV pressure stems from extrinsic forces applied to the LV, mediated by the pericardium and right heart across the interventricular septum.[30] This phenomenon of diastolic ventricular interaction becomes more important as heart size increases (ie, as pericardial space decreases).[31] Even though the LV chamber size usually is normal in HFpEF, total epicardial heart size can be enlarged substantially because of increased atrial size and cardiac hypertrophy, so the pericardial constraint can be relevant.[29] This effect is supported by invasive data from patients who have HFpEF in which the DPVR shifted upwards in patients subjected to exertional stress.[32] In heart failure with low EF, cardiac enlargement in almost all chambers exacerbates pericardial constraint.[31,33] Overfilling of right-sided chambers can increase left-sided pressures via right ventricular (RV)–LV crosstalk as the distending (transmural) pressure that drives LV filling becomes impaired.[34] This mechanism can explain how acute unloading of the right heart paradoxically can increase LV filling and output in patients who have advanced systolic heart failure or cor pulmonale.[33]

AFTERLOAD AND VENTRICULAR–ARTERIAL INTERACTION

Adequate pressure and flow to the body depends both on cardiac performance and on the nature of the vascular load into which it ejects. This load traditionally has been conceived of as equivalent to mean or systolic blood pressure, although this notion can lead to ambiguous interpretations. Unlike isolated muscle (for which the term "afterload" was first defined), where one can fix a constant force during contraction, the intact heart generates varying stress (and pressures) during ejection, and the blood pressure generated is determined as much by the heart's properties as by those of the vasculature.[35] A useful alternative parameter is aortic input impedance, which characterizes the mean and pulsatile properties of the vascular loading circuit and is independent of the heart. Impedance is derived from Fourier analysis of aortic pressure and flow waves,[36,37] traditionally assessed by invasive catheters although noninvasive methods also have been described.

Coupling of impedance to a heart property is mathematically complicated, because impedance is described in the frequency domain (ie, Fourier spectra), and the heart property is described in the time domain. In the early 1980s, however, Sunagawa and colleagues[38,39] developed the parameter effective arterial elastance (Ea), based on LV pressure–volume loop analysis. Ea, like Ees, is measured in units of elastance and can be calculated more easily to study ventricular–arterial interaction. Ea is not a measure of a specific vascular property per se but combines both mean and pulsatile loading (and heart rate influences), providing a lumped parameter reflecting the net impact of this load on the heart. Kelly and colleagues[40] showed that the simple ratio of end-systolic pressure to stroke volume accurately estimates Ea in both hypertensive and normal humans. Graphically Ea is identified by the negative slope running through the end-systolic PV coordinates and EDV at zero pressure (**Fig. 3**). As discussed earlier, LV Ees is determined by the slope of the ESPVR. The Ees reflects chamber contractility but also is influenced by chamber size and remodeling. Knowledge of Ees, Ea, and EDV allows one to predict blood pressure, stroke volume and stroke work, and EF.[8]

Ees and Ea are matched in healthy persons to provide optimal mechanical efficiency in the transfer of blood from the heart to the body, so that the coupling ratio (Ea/Ees) approaches unity.[41] It can be shown mathematically that the EF varies inversely with the Ea/Ees ratio.[8] In systolic heart failure, contractility (Ees) is low, whereas afterload (Ea) usually is high in the setting of vasoconstriction and neurohormonal activation. This condition produces "afterload mismatch" so that the coupling ratio increases, meaning that the EF decreases.[42] With advanced systolic dysfunction, it usually is difficult to increase contractility (Ees) effectively because of limited inotropic reserve, but therapies reducing Ea to very low levels have been extremely useful in optimizing ventricular ejection in such patients.

Conceptualizing systolic heart failure in terms of ventricular–arterial interaction can help explain the

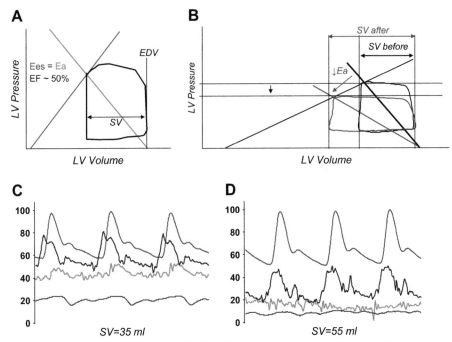

Fig. 3. (*A*) Normal steady-state PV loop. Ea is defined by the negative slope (*green line*) running between the end-systolic PV point and EDV at *P* = 0. In healthy persons, Ees (*red line*) and Ea are matched to maintain optimal coupling and efficiency, with an EF of around 50% to 60% when the volume intercept is near zero. (*B*) In systolic heart failure, the heart is dilated (increased EDV), Ees is low (shallow ESPVR), and the EF is reduced. Acute reduction of Ea with a vasodilator (*red*) leads to a marked 50% increase in stroke volume (SV after) with very little reduction in blood pressure. (*C*) Radial artery (*red*), pulmonary artery (*blue*), pulmonary wedge (*green*), and right atrial (*pink*) pressure versus time in a patient who has dilated cardiomyopathy. There is severe pulmonary arterial and venous hypertension with borderline systemic hypotension. SV, stroke volume. (*D*) The same patient on a high dose (7 μg/kg/min) of sodium nitroprusside. Note the near-normalization of cardiac filling pressures with marked increase in stroke volume (SV), with little change in systolic blood pressure.

clinical response to vasodilator therapy of patients who have dilated cardiomyopathy.[9] **Fig. 3**B shows a typical resting PV loop from such a patient. Because of the shallow slope of the ESPVR (low Ees), there is little change in blood pressure despite a marked improvement in stroke volume for a given dose of vasodilator. **Fig. 3**C and D shows pressure tracings as part of transplant evaluation for a patient who has advanced dilated cardiomyopathy. Filling pressures are high at baseline, pulmonary vascular resistance is prohibitively elevated, and there is systemic hypotension. With the administration of sodium nitroprusside there is marked improvement in cardiac output, filling pressures, and pulmonary vascular resistance and no significant reduction in systolic pressures—all as predicted based on the principals of ventricular–arterial coupling.

Although the coupling ratio is useful for determining stroke volume and the pressure generated during systole, the absolute magnitude of both the numerator and denominator is equally important. In normal aging, systolic hypertension, and renal disease, there are exaggerated increases in both ventricular and vascular stiffness.[8] The stiff ventricle-artery unit creates a "high-gain" system in which there are much larger changes in pressure with relatively little change in stroke volume (**Fig. 4**). This situation is essentially the opposite of that seen in systolic heart failure, where loading changes result in relatively minor alterations in blood pressure, despite more dramatic changes in stroke volume. The importance in ventricular-arterial stiffening becomes most dramatic in many patients who have HFpEF, who can have quite high Ea and Ees.[32] **Fig. 4**B and C shows LV and pulmonary artery pressures from a typical patient who has HFpEF and increased ventricular-arterial stiffness. At rest (see **Fig. 4**B), there is severe systemic and pulmonary artery hypertension. In contrast to the patient who has heart failure and low EF shown in **Fig. 3**, there is a marked hypotensive effect after the administration of a very low dose of nitroprusside (see **Fig. 4**C) with little or no change in stroke volume and cardiac output. In this way, high resting stiffness greatly amplified the change in blood pressure for a given change in preload or afterload while minimizing changes in stroke volume. Increased ventricular-arterial stiffening helps explain the clinical behavior of patients who have HFpEF, who often oscillate between hypertensive crisis and symptomatic hypotension with relatively minor perturbations. Treatments targeting combined stiffening may allow better regulation of PV responses during stress in such patients and are being explored in upcoming clinical trials.[3] **Fig. 5** contrasts the two types of patients schematically, using model-based analyses.

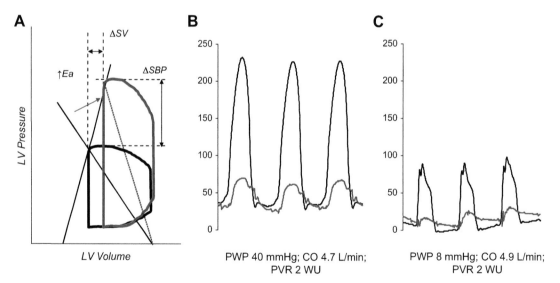

Fig. 4. (*A*) With aging, hypertension, and in HFpEF, ventricular (Ees) and arterial (Ea) stiffness increases. Although the Ea/Ees ratio may remain normal, combined ventricular and vascular stiffening leads to marked fluctuations in blood pressure with relatively small changes in preload or afterload. This condition is in striking contrast to heart failure with low EF (see **Fig. 3**B). (*B*) LV (*black*) and pulmonary artery (*red*) pressure tracings from an 81-year-old woman who has HFpEF demonstrating severe systemic and pulmonary artery hypertension, with markedly elevated LVEDP and wedge pressures (not shown). (*C*) In response to a very low dose of sodium nitroprusside (2 μg), filling pressures normalize, but severe hypotension develops. Note that there is little change in cardiac output (stroke volume) with vasodilation, again in striking contrast to heart failure with reduced EF. CO, cardiac output; PVR, pulmonary vascular resistance; PWP, pulmonary wedge pressure; WU, Wood units.

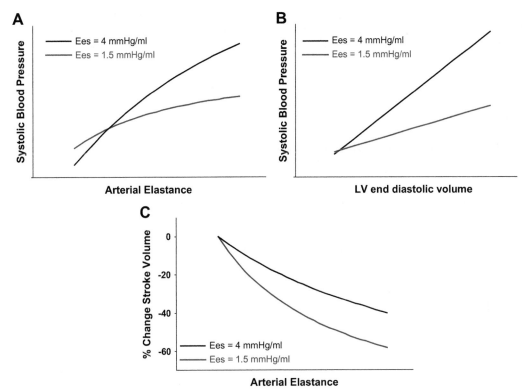

Fig. 5. Increased ventricular systolic stiffness leads to a greater rise in blood pressure for a given increase in (*A*) afterload or (*B*) preload. (*C*) Although isolated increases in afterload lead to a predictable reduction in stroke volume for a given level of contractility, this afterload dependence is more marked in patients who have lower Ees, as seen in patients who have heart failure with reduced EF.

Arterial–ventricular interaction also is important in affecting diastolic processes. Acutely increased vascular load, particularly applied in late ventricular systole,[43] prolongs relaxation in humans and animals.[3,44] Such load dependence becomes more pronounced in heart failure, perhaps related in part to abnormal phosphorylation of sarcomeric proteins. Troponin I phosphorylation by protein kinase A attenuates afterload-induced impairment in early-diastolic relaxation, and mice lacking such phosphorylation sites have enhanced load-dependent relaxation delay.[45] Acute increases in Ea also have been shown to increase LV diastolic stiffness in an aged canine model of HFpEF.[46] LV early-diastolic relaxation varies inversely with net afterload and vascular stiffness in humans with and without hypertensive heart disease[43] and is correlated most closely with pulsatile components, particularly late-systolic load, determined by returning pressure wave reflections and arterial stiffening.

THE RIGHT HEART

Pulmonary hypertension and accompanying right heart dysfunction is increasingly common in

patients who have heart failure, regardless of EF, and potently affect exercise capacity and clinical outcome.[47,48] Pulmonary hypertension generally is defined as a mean pulmonary arterial pressure higher than 25 mm Hg at rest (30 mm Hg with exercise), whereas pulmonary arterial hypertension (ie, pulmonary vascular disease) further requires an elevated pulmonary vascular resistance while maintaining a normal pulmonary capillary wedge pressure.[49] The presence of pulmonary vascular resistance and the ability to reduce it with vasodilators are used commonly to establish eligibility for cardiac transplantation. Drug testing uses nitric oxide donators or milrinone and, more recently, the phosphodiesterase 5 inhibitor sildenafil and the natriuretic peptide nesiritide.[50] Although pulmonary artery pressures can be estimated by echo-Doppler methods, invasive assessment is required for definitive diagnosis and to guide treatment decisions.[49]

With the wide use of echo-Doppler cardiography, pulmonary hypertension now is being recognized increasingly, particularly among the older patients presenting with dypsnea.[51] The prevalence of suspected idiopathic pulmonary hypertension of the elderly is increasing, and in many cases the condition may be a forme fruste of HFpEF. Recent studies have found that these patients tend to have higher left heart filling pressures than younger patients who have more traditional isolated pulmonary arterial hypertension.[51] Invasive hemodynamic assessment in the catheterization laboratory can be extremely useful in evaluating such patients, many of whom complain of exertional dyspnea and whose symptoms could be explained by multiple, potentially competing causes (eg, diastolic dysfunction, pulmonary vascular disease, obesity, deconditioning, and others). Interpreting elevated pulmonary wedge pressures in such patients often is difficult, because in the setting of right heart and left atrial enlargement enhanced extrinsic pressure may be applied via the pericardium.[31]

Compared with the left side, the assessment of right ventricular function remains fairly primitive. Standard two-dimensional echocardiographic views often are difficult to standardize to provide reproducible parameters, and the shape of the RV limits the use of simple geometric models to derive accurate volumetric data. As with the LV, RV pressures are not determined exclusively by the ventricle or vasculature but rather result from the dynamic interaction of the two. The RV PV loop normally is triangular, reflecting the lower resistive load and relatively higher compliance of the pulmonary vascular circuit, although it becomes more rectangular (like the LV) in patients who have pulmonary hypertension (perhaps making application of standard LV approaches and the assumptions behind them more justified in this setting). Assessment of RV diastolic stiffness is quite rare in the literature and is affected greatly by pericardial restraint and biventricular remodeling. RV vascular impedance consists of mean pulmonary resistance, the proximal stiffness of pulmonary conduit arteries, characteristic impedance, distal vascular compliance, and reflected waves. There now is renewed interest in how these properties of impedance can impose late-systolic loads on the RV[52] (much as they do on the LV), impacting RV remodeling, relaxation delay, and inefficiency.

The importance of the right heart–pulmonary vascular interaction on symptoms in chronic heart failure is appreciated increasingly. Traditional vasodilators used to treat heart failure (eg, converting enzyme inhibitors and angiotensin receptor blockers) tend to have less effect on the pulmonary circuit. Treatments used to target the pulmonary vasculature, such as prostacyclin and endothelin antagonists, also have systemic effects and have not yet been evaluated larger-scale

clinical trials in patients who have predominantly left-sided heart failure. Phosphodiesterase inhibitors such as sildenafil reduce pulmonary vascular resistance while having mild systemic vascular effects, and these drugs are helping elucidate RV-pulmonary pathophysiology in heart failure. In an elegant series of recent studies performed in humans who had primary left-sided systolic heart failure, sildenafil acutely and chronically reduced pulmonary resistance, correlating with enhanced exercise capacity, without much systemic change.[53,54] In another study, investigators found sildenafil improved endothelial function (flow-mediated dilation) in addition to reducing pulmonary resistance, and this improvement also was coupled with improved exercise capacity.[55] Given the lack of obvious left-sided heart or arterial resistive effects, these studies highlight the importance of enhancing pulmonary vascular throughput and normal vasodilator reserve in patients who have heart failure.

INVASIVE HEMODYNAMICS: A RE-EMERGING ROLE IN THE EVALUATION OF PATIENTS WHO HAVE POSSIBLE HEART FAILURE AND PRESERVED EJECTION FRACTION

Most cardiologists are fairly confident in making the diagnosis of heart failure when a patient who has severe LV enlargement and an EF of 25% presents with dyspnea, but a significant group of patients present with exertional dyspnea, clinical euvolemia (or only mild hypervolemia), and a normal EF. The differential diagnosis is fairly broad, including noncardiac causes (deconditioning, obesity, anemia, and other possibilities) and a variety of cardiogenic sources. These conditions may include valvular disease, isolated right heart failure, pulmonary vascular disease, constrictive pericarditis, restrictive cardiomyopathy, or "garden variety" HFpEF. The correct diagnosis often can be made from the combination of physical examination, comprehensive echo-Doppler evaluation, and plasma natriuretic peptide levels. In many patients, particularly the elderly, the picture is not so clear, because diastolic dysfunction seen on echo-Doppler imaging is common in this cohort,[21] and natriuretic peptide levels may be mildly elevated even in the absence of true heart failure.[56]

Invasive hemodynamic assessment in the catheterization laboratory can be clinically useful in these cases. **Fig. 6** shows hemodynamics from an 80-year-old woman who has class II-III dyspnea, normal EF, mild diastolic dysfunction, and mild to moderate pulmonary hypertension on echocardiogram. Filling pressures are normal at

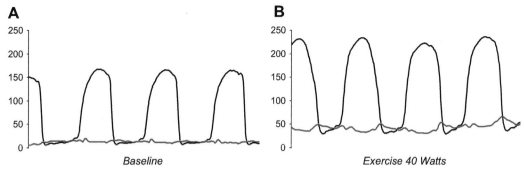

Fig. 6. (*A*) LV (*black*) and pulmonary wedge (*red*) pressures at rest in a patient who has symptoms of New York Heart Association class II-III dyspnea and normal LV size and function on echocardiogram. Despite mild to moderate systemic hypertension, cardiac filling pressures are normal, arguing against heart failure. (*B*) With low-level (40 W) supine exercise in the catheterization laboratory, there is a dramatic increase in cardiac filling pressures (to 45–50 mm Hg) associated with significant dyspnea, suggesting that HFpEF indeed is the cause of the patient's symptoms.

rest (see **Fig. 6**A), suggesting that the patient's symptoms may not be related to heart failure. Supine exercise at low workload (see **Fig. 6**B), however, reveals a marked increase in cardiac filling pressures associated with severe symptoms of dyspnea. Pulmonary artery pressures increase in proportion to the increase in pulmonary wedge, indicating that the patient's symptoms probably are caused primarily by HFpEF. Other patients may show filling pressures and cardiac output that are normal both at rest and at maximal workload, arguing against a diagnosis of HFpEF. Finally, others develop pulmonary arterial hypertension with exercise in the absence of an increase in left heart filling pressures, identifying a more isolated lesion at the level of the pulmonary vasculature. In practice, individual patients may embody any of these conditions or, more commonly, present with some combination of all three, and future research is required to understand how best to treat patients who have each type of response.

Patients who have had cardiac surgery or radiation therapy may present months to years later with predominant right-sided heart failure, and high-fidelity cardiac catheterization focusing on relationships between intrathoracic–intracardiac pressure dissociation and diastolic ventricular interaction can identify whether symptoms are caused predominantly by constrictive physiology, valvular disease, or restrictive cardiomyopathy.[57,58] Administration of arterial vasodilators such as nitroprusside can be useful to determine whether elevated filling pressures are caused by a partially load-dependent process, such as diastolic dysfunction, or an irreversible myopathic process, such as restrictive cardiomyopathy.

Right heart catheterization can be useful in the management of patients who have acute decompensated heart failure, particularly in the setting of right-sided congestion, low cardiac output, and worsening renal function, when central hemodynamic status remains uncertain. In addition, central hemodynamics may provide independent prognostic value in patients who have heart failure. Each of these topics is discussed elsewhere in this issue.

The time course of ventricular stiffening (ie, elastance varying over time, long a bio-engineering concept[59] but with little apparent interest to physicians) could become clinically important in the near future. Novel therapies targeting myofilament calcium sensitivity and/or the filaments (activators) themselves to increase force generation without altering activator calcium or stimulating cAMP/ protein kinase A (PKA) cascades are in development.[60] Although phosphorylation of myosin-binding protein C augments early dP/dt_{max} downstream of β-adrenergic stimulation,[4] sensitizers/activators do not work in this manner. Instead of affecting isovolumic contraction, these drugs often enhance myocardial stiffening (elastance), prolonging the time for elastance to reach its peak and thus making the ejection time longer. The difference in mechanisms is not easily discerned from traditional methods of analysis but is shown readily by the elastance curves. **Fig. 7** shows a schematic of such curves comparing the effects of a beta-agonist to a Ca^{2+}-sensitizer. The beta-agonist increases the rate of rise and fall of myocardial stiffening but shortens systole. In contrast, the sensitizer has little effect on the rates of rise and fall but prolongs ejection. The lure of sensitizers is their potential to provide inotropy without the increases in heart rate, risk of arrhythmia, or metabolic demand seen with traditional cAMP/PKA-mediated agonists. Such drugs are being developed, so this type of hemodynamic

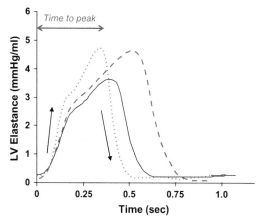

Fig. 7. Time varying elastance curves obtained at baseline (*solid line*), after β-adrenergic stimulation (*dotted line*), and in response to an agent that enhances myofilament calcium sensitivity (*dashed line*). Although the calcium sensitizer has less effect on the early rise in elastance, there is an increase in the time to peak elastance and systolic duration. See text for details.

analysis, or a simplified version of it, ultimately may provide ways to index and follow the effects of these drugs in individual patients.

SUMMARY

A few years after fading from the forefront of cardiology, interest in cardiovascular hemodynamics is returning, especially as newer devices are developed that help measure these parameters in patients chronically. Invasive assessment of cardiovascular properties provides greater insight into the mechanisms of disease in disorders such as HFpEF and can explain how patients who have different forms of heart failure respond to various therapies or to certain forms of stress. This information may be useful for treating individual patients and in understanding group differences and treatment effects. Invasive hemodynamic assessment remains the reference standard for assessing systolic and diastolic function and ventricular–arterial interaction and can allow more definitive diagnosis of heart failure, especially in patients where the diagnosis of HF that is based upon clinical and oninvasive evaluation alone remains uncertain.

REFERENCES

1. Kass DA, Maughan WL, Guo ZM, et al. Comparative influence of load versus inotropic states on indexes of ventricular contractility: experimental and theoretical analysis based on pressure-volume relationships. Circulation 1987;76(6):1422–36.

2. Hunt SA, Abraham WT, Chin MH, et al. ACC/AHA 2005 guideline update for the diagnosis and management of chronic heart failure in the adult: a report of the American College of Cardiology/ American Heart Association Task Force on Practice Guidelines (Writing Committee to Update the 2001 Guidelines for the Evaluation and Management of Heart Failure): developed in collaboration with the American College of Chest Physicians and the International Society for Heart and Lung Transplantation: endorsed by the Heart Rhythm Society. Circulation 2005;112(12):e154–235.

3. Borlaug BA, Kass DA. Mechanisms of diastolic dysfunction in heart failure. Trends Cardiovasc Med 2006;16(8):273–9.

4. Nagayama T, Takimoto E, Sadayappan S, et al. Control of in vivo left ventricular [correction] contraction/relaxation kinetics by myosin binding protein C: protein kinase A phosphorylation dependent and independent regulation. Circulation 2007;116(21): 2399–408.

5. Spragg DD, Kass DA. Pathobiology of left ventricular dyssynchrony and resynchronization. Prog Cardiovasc Dis 2006;49(1):26–41.

6. Baicu CF, Zile MR, Aurigemma GP, et al. Left ventricular systolic performance, function, and contractility in patients with diastolic heart failure. Circulation 2005;111(18):2306–12.

7. Suga H, Sagawa K. Instantaneous pressure-volume relationships and their ratio in the excised, supported canine left ventricle. Circ Res 1974;35(1): 117–26.

8. Borlaug BA, Kass DA. Ventricular-vascular interaction in heart failure. Heart Fail Clin 2008;4(1):23–36.

9. Kass DA, Maughan WL. From 'Emax' to pressure-volume relations: a broader view. Circulation 1988; 77(6):1203–12.

10. Chen CH, Fetics B, Nevo E, et al. Noninvasive single-beat determination of left ventricular end-systolic elastance in humans. J Am Coll Cardiol 2001;38(7):2028–34.

11. Lee WS, Huang WP, Yu WC, et al. Estimation of preload recruitable stroke work relationship by a single-beat technique in humans. Am J Physiol Heart Circ Physiol 2003;284(2):H744–50.

12. Borlaug BA, Melenovsky V, Marhin T, et al. Sildenafil inhibits beta-adrenergic-stimulated cardiac contractility in humans. Circulation 2005;112(17): 2642–9.

13. Redfield MM, Jacobsen SJ, Borlaug BA, et al. Age- and gender-related ventricular-vascular stiffening: a community-based study. Circulation 2005; 112(15):2254–62.

14. Lam CS, Roger VL, Rodeheffer RJ, et al. Cardiac structure and ventricular-vascular function in

persons with heart failure and preserved ejection fraction from olmsted county, Minnesota. Circulation 2007;115(15):1982–90.

15. Glower DD, Spratt JA, Snow ND, et al. Linearity of the Frank-Starling relationship in the intact heart: the concept of preload recruitable stroke work. Circulation 1985;71(5):994–1009.

16. Kass DA, Beyar R. Evaluation of contractile state by maximal ventricular power divided by the square of end-diastolic volume. Circulation 1991; 84(4):1698–708.

17. Sharir T, Feldman MD, Haber H, et al. Ventricular systolic assessment in patients with dilated cardiomyopathy by preload-adjusted maximal power. Validation and noninvasive application. Circulation 1994;89(5):2045–53.

18. Senzaki H, Fetics B, Chen CH, et al. Comparison of ventricular pressure relaxation assessments in human heart failure: quantitative influence on load and drug sensitivity analysis. J Am Coll Cardiol 1999;34(5):1529–36.

19. Matsubara H, Takaki M, Yasuhara S, et al. Logistic time constant of isovolumic relaxation pressure-time curve in the canine left ventricle. Better alternative to exponential time constant. Circulation 1995; 92(8):2318–26.

20. Chung CS, Kovacs SJ. Physical determinants of left ventricular isovolumic pressure decline: model prediction with in vivo validation. Am J Physiol Heart Circ Physiol 2008;294(4):H1589–96.

21. Redfield MM, Jacobsen SJ, Burnett JC Jr, et al. Burden of systolic and diastolic ventricular dysfunction in the community: appreciating the scope of the heart failure epidemic. JAMA 2003;289(2):194–202.

22. Glantz SA, Parmley WW. Factors which affect the diastolic pressure-volume curve. Circ Res 1978; 42(2):171–80.

23. Oh JK, Hatle L, Tajik AJ, et al. Diastolic heart failure can be diagnosed by comprehensive two-dimensional and Doppler echocardiography. J Am Coll Cardiol 2006;47(3):500–6.

24. Kass DA. Assessment of diastolic dysfunction. Invasive modalities. Cardiol Clin 2000;18(3):571–86.

25. Pak PH, Maughan L, Baughman KL, et al. Marked discordance between dynamic and passive diastolic pressure-volume relations in idiopathic hypertrophic cardiomyopathy. Circulation 1996;94(1):52–60.

26. Zile MR, Baicu CF, Gaasch WH. Diastolic heart failure–abnormalities in active relaxation and passive stiffness of the left ventricle. N Engl J Med 2004;350(19):1953–9.

27. Westermann D, Kasner M, Steendijk P, et al. Role of left ventricular stiffness in heart failure with normal ejection fraction. Circulation 2008;117(16):2051–60.

28. Maurer MS, Burkhoff D, Fried LP, et al. Ventricular structure and function in hypertensive participants with heart failure and a normal ejection fraction:

the Cardiovascular Health Study. J Am Coll Cardiol 2007;49(9):972–81.

29. Melenovsky V, Borlaug BA, Rosen B, et al. Cardiovascular features of heart failure with preserved ejection fraction versus nonfailing hypertensive left ventricular hypertrophy in the urban Baltimore community: the role of atrial remodeling/dysfunction. J Am Coll Cardiol 2007;49(2):198–207.

30. Dauterman K, Pak PH, Maughan WL, et al. Contribution of external forces to left ventricular diastolic pressure. Implications for the clinical use of the Starling law. Ann Intern Med 1995;122(10):737–42.

31. Frenneaux M, Williams L. Ventricular-arterial and ventricular-ventricular interactions and their relevance to diastolic filling. Prog Cardiovasc Dis 2007;49(4):252–62.

32. Kawaguchi M, Hay I, Fetics B, et al. Combined ventricular systolic and arterial stiffening in patients with heart failure and preserved ejection fraction: implications for systolic and diastolic reserve limitations. Circulation 2003;107(5):714–20.

33. Atherton JJ, Moore TD, Lele SS, et al. Diastolic ventricular interaction in chronic heart failure. Lancet 1997;349(9067):1720–4.

34. Moore TD, Frenneaux MP, Sas R, et al. Ventricular interaction and external constraint account for decreased stroke work during volume loading in CHF. Am J Physiol Heart Circ Physiol 2001;281(6): H2385–91.

35. Kass DA, Kelly RP. Ventriculo-arterial coupling: concepts, assumptions, and applications. Ann Biomed Eng 1992;20(1):41–62.

36. Milnor WR. Arterial impedance as ventricular afterload. Circ Res 1975;36(5):565–70.

37. Murgo JP, Westerhof N, Giolma JP, et al. Aortic input impedance in normal man: relationship to pressure wave forms. Circulation 1980;62(1):105–16.

38. Sunagawa K, Maughan WL, Burkhoff D, et al. Left ventricular interaction with arterial load studied in isolated canine ventricle. Am J Physiol 1983; 245(5 Pt 1):H773–80.

39. Sunagawa K, Maughan WL, Sagawa K. Optimal arterial resistance for the maximal stroke work studied in isolated canine left ventricle. Circ Res 1985;56(4):586–95.

40. Kelly RP, Ting CT, Yang TM, et al. Effective arterial elastance as index of arterial vascular load in humans. Circulation 1992;86(2):513–21.

41. De Tombe PP, Jones S, Burkhoff D, et al. Ventricular stroke work and efficiency both remain nearly optimal despite altered vascular loading. Am J Physiol 1993;264(6 Pt 2):H1817–24.

42. Asanoi H, Sasayama S, Kameyama T. Ventriculoarterial coupling in normal and failing heart in humans. Circ Res 1989;65(2):483–93.

43. Borlaug BA, Melenovsky V, Redfield MM, et al. Impact of arterial load and loading sequence on

left ventricular tissue velocities in humans. J Am Coll Cardiol 2007;50(16):1570–7.

44. Gillebert TC, Leite-Moreira AF, De Hert SG. Load dependent diastolic dysfunction in heart failure. Heart Fail Rev 2000;5(4):345–55.

45. Bilchick KC, Duncan JG, Ravi R, et al. Heart failure-associated alterations in troponin I phosphorylation impair ventricular relaxation-afterload and force-frequency responses and systolic function. Am J Physiol Heart Circ Physiol 2007;292(1):H318–25.

46. Shapiro BP, Lam CS, Patel JB, et al. Acute and chronic ventricular-arterial coupling in systole and diastole. Insights from an elderly hypertensive model. Hypertension 2007;50(3):503–11.

47. Haddad F, Doyle R, Murphy DJ, et al. Right ventricular function in cardiovascular disease, part II: pathophysiology, clinical importance, and management of right ventricular failure. Circulation 2008;117(13):1717–31.

48. Kjaergaard J, Akkan D, Iversen KK, et al. Prognostic importance of pulmonary hypertension in patients with heart failure. Am J Cardiol 2007;99(8):1146–50.

49. McGoon M, Gutterman D, Steen V, et al. Screening, early detection, and diagnosis of pulmonary arterial hypertension: ACCP evidence-based clinical practice guidelines. Chest 2004;126(1 Suppl):14S–34S.

50. Alaeddini J, Uber PA, Park MH, et al. Efficacy and safety of sildenafil in the evaluation of pulmonary hypertension in severe heart failure. Am J Cardiol 2004;94(11):1475–7.

51. Shapiro BP, McGoon MD, Redfield MM. Unexplained pulmonary hypertension in elderly patients. Chest 2007;131(1):94–100.

52. Kussmaul WG 3rd, Altschuler JA, Matthai WH, et al. Right ventricular-vascular interaction in congestive heart failure. Importance of low-frequency impedance. Circulation 1993;88(3):1010–5.

53. Lepore JJ, Maroo A, Bigatello LM, et al. Hemodynamic effects of sildenafil in patients with congestive heart failure and pulmonary hypertension: combined administration with inhaled nitric oxide. Chest 2005;127(5):1647–53.

54. Lewis GD, Lachmann J, Camuso J, et al. Sildenafil improves exercise hemodynamics and oxygen uptake in patients with systolic heart failure. Circulation 2007;115(1):59–66.

55. Guazzi M, Samaja M, Arena R, et al. Long-term use of sildenafil in the therapeutic management of heart failure. J Am Coll Cardiol 2007;50(22):2136–44.

56. Costello-Boerrigter LC, Boerrigter G, Redfield MM, et al. Amino-terminal pro-B-type natriuretic peptide and B-type natriuretic peptide in the general community: determinants and detection of left ventricular dysfunction. J Am Coll Cardiol 2006;47(2):345–53.

57. Hurrell DG, Nishimura RA, Higano ST, et al. Value of dynamic respiratory changes in left and right ventricular pressures for the diagnosis of constrictive pericarditis. Circulation 1996;93(11):2007–13.

58. Talreja DR, Nishimura RA, Oh JK, et al. Constrictive pericarditis in the modern era: novel criteria for diagnosis in the cardiac catheterization laboratory. J Am Coll Cardiol 2008;51(3):315–9.

59. Suga H, Sagawa K, Demer L. Determinants of instantaneous pressure in canine left ventricle. Time and volume specification. Circ Res 1980;46(2):256–63.

60. Kass DA, Solaro RJ. Mechanisms and use of calcium-sensitizing agents in the failing heart. Circulation 2006;113(2):305–15.

Role of the Pulmonary Artery Catheter in Diagnosis and Management of Heart Failure

Rami Kahwash, MD[a],*, Carl V. Leier, MD[a],
Leslie Miller, MD[b,c]

KEYWORDS

- Decompensated heart failure • Pulmonary artery catheter
- Swan-Ganz catheter • Congestive heart failure
- Management of heart failure

Almost 4 decades have passed since the introduction of the balloon-tipped, flow-directed pulmonary artery catheter (PAC) by Swan and colleagues.[1] This technical achievement transformed the pulmonary artery catheter from a laboratory device into a practical bedside tool capable of providing continuous central hemodynamic monitoring. The PAC, once defined as "the cornerstone of the intensive care units" and regarded as an important management tool, has faced noteworthy scrutiny in the past 2 decades. Starting in the late 1980s, several reports raised concern about the actual impact of pulmonary artery catheter use on improving clinical outcomes.[2–4] Concerns intensified after a large retrospective observational trial suggested possible harm associated with the use of PAC.[5,6] Several prospective studies were then performed to evaluate the outcomes of PAC use in a variety of acute medical and surgical conditions,[7–12] including decompensated chronic heart failure.[13] Despite differences in study designs and heterogeneities of studied populations, results from these randomized clinical trials have consistently shown lack of any measurable outcomes benefit from the routine use of PACs in critically ill patients. Consequently, PACs in clinical practice have undergone a steep decline in use. Between 1993 and 2004, PAC use has decreased by up to 65% for all medical admissions in many institutions, with the sharpest decline seen in the management of acute myocardial infarction (81%), acute respiratory failure (76%), and septicemia (54%) **(Fig. 1)**.[14]

This article addresses the role of PACs in the diagnosis and management of heart failure, the Evaluation Study of Congestive Heart Failure and Pulmonary Artery Catheterization Effectiveness (ESCAPE) trial and registry, the impact of ESCAPE and related studies on the practical management of heart failure, and the general indications for PAC application in current clinical practice.

TECHNICAL EVOLUTION OF THE PULMONARY ARTERY CATHETER

The PAC is an interesting tool that enjoyed an exciting journey from the time it was discovered up to current times. By act of an inadvertent

---

This article originally appeared in *Heart Failure Clinics*, volume 5, number 2.

[a] Davis Heart/Lung Research Institute, Columbus, OH, USA
[b] Washington Hospital Center, Washington, DC, USA
[c] Georgetown University Hospital, Washington, DC, USA
* Corresponding author. Department of Cardiovascular Medicine, The Ohio State University, Davis Heart/Lung Research Institute, 473 West 12th Avenue, Columbus, OH 43210.
E-mail address: rami.kahwash@osumc.edu

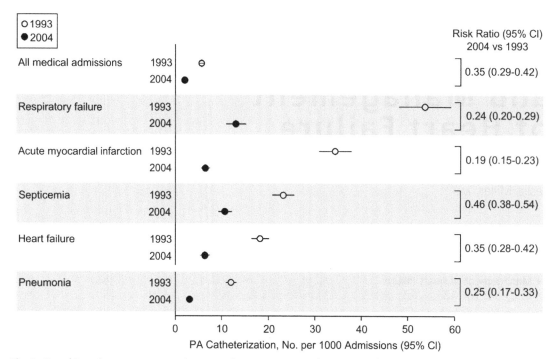

Fig. 1. Trend in pulmonary artery catheter use between 1993 and 2004 according to pre-identified diagnoses. PA, pulmonary artery; CI, confidence intervals. (*From* Wiener RS, Welch HG Trends in the use of the pulmonary artery catheter in the United States, 1993–2004. JAMA 2007;298:423–9; with permission.)

exploration, Forssmann was first to establish the concept of right heart catheterization in 1929.[15] With the intent to deliver drugs directly into the heart, Forssmann advanced a ureteral catheter into his own heart by accessing an "elbow vein" (likely antecubital), and confirmed the presence of the catheter's tip in his right atrium with an x-ray image; this event is regarded by many as the birth of cardiovascular catheterization.

About a decade later, Cournand and Richards[16–18] expanded the use of the right heart catheter to measure right heart pressures and cardiac output. Their work also provided a better understanding of cardiopulmonary hemodynamics and gas exchange. In 1956, Forssmann, Cournand, and Richards received the Nobel Prize in Medicine for their work in the development of the PAC. Although measurement of pulmonary capillary wedge pressure was first described in 1949 by Hellems and colleagues,[19] the link between the pulmonary wedge pressure and the left atrial pressure, however, was established in 1954 by Connolly and colleagues.[20]

After its introduction in the mid 1940s, the PAC remained investigational and confined to the catheterization laboratories for research purposes and limited clinical diagnoses. Over the following years, two major challenges remained to be solved for the PAC: first, the ability to obtain continuous

recordings of human central hemodynamics; and second, transferring the use of the PAC from the research and diagnostic laboratories to the patient's bedside. In 1970, both challenges were achieved by H.J.C. Swan and colleagues,[1] who added a balloon to the catheter tip of the standard PAC, allowing blood flow–directed movement and positioning. This novel idea has indeed shaped the future of this device. Balloon-tipped PACs not only provided clinicians with the ease and safety of bedside placement via floatation of the catheter tip upstream, it enabled them to measure right atrial pressure and PA pressure continuously and pulmonary capillary wedge pressure intermittently via inflation and deflation of the balloon. About a year later, W. Ganz and colleagues[21] added a thermistor to the tip of the catheter allowing direct measurement of cardiac output by thermodilution technique (using temperature as the indicator). For their renowned contribution to the advancement of this clinical tool, medical communities worldwide began to refer to the PAC as the "Swan-Ganz catheter."

CLINICAL TRIALS THAT SHAPED THE HISTORY OF THE PULMONARY ARTERY CATHETER

When Swan and Ganz launched their balloon-tipped, flow-directed PAC in 1970, the use of

PACs expanded considerably and gained in popularity. Physicians now had a means to perform continuous monitoring of central hemodynamics (eg, pulmonary artery pressure, pulmonary wedge pressure, and cardiac output). PAC use was initially directed at the care of patients with acute myocardial infarction, shock, or heart failure, and later extended to surgical units, despite the lack of any solid scientific evidence to support its widespread clinical application. In 1976, the Medical Device Amendments were added to the Food, Drug, and Cosmetic Act of 1938, establishing the branch for Devices and Radiological Health of the Food and Drug Administration (FDA); the intent was to evaluate and regulate the application of medical devices in clinical practice. However, because of some exceptions in rulings, the PAC escaped intense investigation and scrutiny early in its development and its use then proceeded without strict regulation.

In the mid 1970s, reports by Forrester and colleagues[22,23] supported the regular application of PACs in patients with myocardial infarction complicated by hemodynamic instability. Their conclusions were complemented by Rao and colleagues[24] who retrospectively investigated the impact of PACs on reducing perioperative mortality between 1973 and 1976 and prospectively between 1977 and 1982; they found a significant decrease in the rate of perioperative myocardial infarction, from 7.7% to 1.9% (P<.005) in patients who required PACs to guide therapy. Additional favorable reports followed and contributed to the surge in the popularity of this device over the ensuing 20 years.[25,26]

The golden era for PACs, however, was disrupted by the first large negative study published in 1987 by Gore and colleagues.[5] Although the study was a retrospective look, the results indicated that PAC use may be associated with an increased mortality in patients hospitalized for acute myocardial infarction complicated by congestive heart failure (CHF), hypotension, and/or cardiogenic shock. In their retrospective investigation of 3263 patients, hospital mortality was 44.8% in heart failure patients selected to be managed with a PAC compared with 25.3% in those who did not receive a PAC (P<.001). Among hypotensive patients, PAC use was associated with a 48.3% mortality compared with 32.2% in the non-PAC hypotensive group (P<.001). Shock patients did poorly in both groups with mortality of 74.4% in the PAC group and 79.1% in the non-PAC group (not different statistically). PAC use was also associated with a longer duration of hospitalization. Among survivors at hospital discharge, 5-year mortality was the same in both groups. This study

has been heavily criticized for its retrospective chart review, case control design, and lack of risk adjustment. Furthermore, it is hard to identify one intervention (PAC use) as causal in such high-risk patients. The accompanying editorial by Robin,[6] encouraged more rigorous investigation in the use of PACs in clinical practice. At that point in time, 20% to 43% of all patients admitted to critical care units underwent placement of PACs during their stay.[5,27]

Within a decade, prospective studies regarding PAC use started to unfold. Connors and colleagues[7] prospectively studied the relationship between PACs and outcomes (mortality and length of stay) and cost of care in critically ill patients. Results showed that patients managed with PACs within 24 hours of admission had a significantly increased 30-day mortality (odds ratio [OR]: 1.24; 95% confidence interval [CI], 1.03-1.49), higher hospital costs, and longer length of stay. This study and the accompanying editorial by Dalen and Bone,[28] were among those that led the Heart, Lung, and Blood Institute of the National Institutes of Health to call for workshops to further examine the clinical application of PAC use in all areas of clinical medicine. From there, the Evaluation Study of Congestive Heart Failure and Pulmonary Artery catheterization Effectiveness (ESCAPE) Trial[29] was developed and conducted as the first prospective randomized trial designed to assess the benefits of PAC use in managing patients with advanced symptomatic congestive heart failure.

PULMONARY ARTERY CATHETERS IN HEART FAILURE POPULATIONS
Basic Management Concepts in the Pre-Evaluation Study of Congestive Heart Failure and Pulmonary Artery Catheterization Effectiveness Era

Before we discuss ESCAPE, it is important to address some of the approaches to managing decompensated heart failure in the pre-ESCAPE trial era. The concept of "tailored therapy" was developed for patients with decompensated heart failure. With the ultimate goal of relieving the symptoms of congestion and volume overload, tailored therapy is a strategy that involves using PAC-derived hemodynamic data to guide therapy and achieve optimal hemodynamic responses to administered dosing of intravenous agents (eg, nitroprusside, nitroglycerin); thereafter, oral medications were adjusted to match the optimal response. Proponents of this approach have advocated that optimal hemodynamics via PAC-monitored selection of the best drugs (and at the most appropriate doses) would lead to optimal clinical outcomes. Preliminary studies showed that tailored therapy may improve cardiac performance, functional status, and heart failure symptoms and lead to better outcomes in patients with lower filling pressures at discharge.[30–32] The lack of a randomized, parallel non-PAC control arm was a major limitation of these studies.

The Evaluation Study of Congestive Heart Failure and Pulmonary Artery Catheterization Effectiveness Trial and Registry

The ESCAPE trial[13] was the first prospectively randomized, controlled multicenter trial designed to evaluate the use of the PAC in hospitalized patients with advanced heart failure. The study intent was to determine whether the addition of PAC-guided therapy to clinical assessment would further enhance outcomes (reduce mortality and hospitalizations) over therapy guided by clinical assessment alone in patients with advanced symptomatic heart failure. A total of 26 study centers with very experienced heart failure specialists in the United States and Canada participated in this trial between 2000 and 2003. A total of 433 patients were enrolled with goals of relieving clinical congestion and improving symptoms in both treatment groups. Patients were randomly assigned to the clinical assessment group, for which therapeutic decisions were guided by clinical assessment alone or to the pulmonary artery catheter group, for which therapy was guided by clinical assessment in addition to central hemodynamic data provided by the PAC. Entry criteria included severely symptomatic heart failure and overt signs of congestion, for which PAC use was felt to be beneficial for management; however, patients still had to be stable enough so that PAC management would not be absolutely necessary or mandatory. Patients with advanced renal failure and those who required intravenous inotropic agents for clinical stabilization were excluded from the trial. The overall target of therapy in both groups was the resolution of signs and symptoms of clinical congestion, but in the PAC group, a pulmonary artery capillary wedge pressure of 15 mm Hg or less and right atrial pressure of 8 mm Hg or less were also targeted. The primary trial end point was the total number of days alive out of the hospital in the first 6 months after enrollment. Secondary end points included exercise tolerance, quality of life, and echocardiographic measurements.

Both groups experienced improvement in symptoms and signs of congestion, and there was no statistical difference in the primary end point. The number of days alive out of the hospital in the first 6 months between the clinical assessment and the PAC group were 133 days and 135 days respectively, with a hazard ratio of 1.00 (95% CI: 0.82-1.21) (**Fig. 2**). Mortality at 6 months did not statistically differ between the two groups as well (10% vs 9%, respectively, OR: 1.26, 95% CI: 0.78–2.03). Subgroup analyses also generally yielded neutral results when looking at pre-specified factors (**Fig. 3**). Secondary end point analyses revealed a favorable effect on time trade-off for the PAC group, and a trend toward improvement in 6-minute walk during the index hospitalization in the PAC group; however, this trend did not quite reach statistical significance. On the other hand, adverse events were higher in the PAC group (21.9% vs 11.5%, $P = .04$). PAC-related adverse events occurred in nine patients in the PAC group compared with one patient in the clinical assessment group who ended up receiving a PAC later. Most PAC-related adverse events were infection (four patients), with no death linked directly to placement of a PAC.

The ESCAPE trial is a landmark study, being the first large, prospectively randomized, controlled investigation that specifically evaluated the use of PACs in patients with symptomatic, advanced heart failure. As can be readily discerned, the results of the ESCAPE trial do not support the

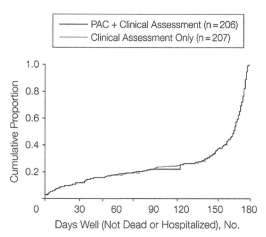

Fig. 2. Cumulative primary end point (days alive and out of hospital) in the ESCAPE trial. Note that the curves overlap for the two treatment groups, pulmonary artery catheter (PAC) plus clinical assessment versus clinical assessment alone. n and NO, number. (*From* Binanay C, Califf RM, Hasselblad V, et al. ESCAPE Investigators and ESCAPE Study Coordinators. Evaluation study of congestive heart failure and pulmonary artery catheterization effectiveness: The ESCAPE Trial. JAMA 2005;294(13):1625–33; with permission.)

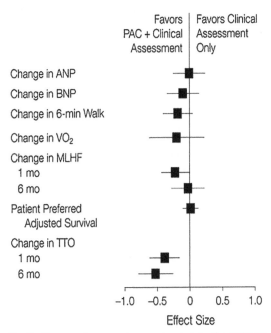

Fig. 3. Changes in secondary end points in the ESCAPE trial. ANP, atrial natriuretic peptide; BNP, brain natriuretic peptide; VO₂, peak oxygen consumption; MLHF, Minnesota Living with Heart Failure questionnaire; TTO, time trade-off score. (*From* Binanay C, Califf RM, Hasselblad V, et al. ESCAPE Investigators and ESCAPE Study Coordinators. Evaluation study of congestive heart failure and pulmonary artery catheterization effectiveness: The ESCAPE Trial. JAMA 2005;294:1625–33; with permission.)

regular use of pulmonary artery catheter in guiding therapy of patients hospitalized with advanced, symptomatic heart failure. The neutral ESCAPE results are in general agreement with prior reports that included heart failure subgroups among their study populations.[7,8]

Several points merit consideration before we finalize conclusions from the ESCAPE trial. First, ESCAPE enrolled patients with symptomatic advanced heart failure, for whom clinical management guided by clinical assessment alone was felt reasonably sufficient by experienced heart failure physicians. In other words, patients whose management absolutely required a PAC were actually excluded from the study. Thus, generalization of the ESCAPE trial results to all heart failure patients, regardless of their clinical profile and status should be avoided. Second, the ESCAPE trial did not include patients with cardiogenic shock, or patients being evaluated for mechanical assist devices or urgent heart transplantation. Third, the ESCAPE trial fell short of providing guidelines to choose and guide therapy

based on the central hemodynamic data provided by PAC use. The lack of mandated algorithms likely created wide differences among treating physicians in the selection and sequence of therapies (and dosing) for each patient. The effect of this heterogeneous approach on the study outcome is unknown. Finally, the ESCAPE investigators were highly experienced heart failure physicians with outstanding clinical experience and an extraordinary ability to implement their clinical skills in complex patient management. The diminished added benefits of a PAC-guided strategy over therapy guided by their clinical assessment alone may, in part, be the result of a superb performance in the clinical assessment arm (control group). In fact, the rate of PAC-related complications was lower in higher enrollment centers, suggesting the role and impact of skilled physicians in the ESCAPE outcomes.

Could management with PACs actually alter prognosis or is PAC use simply a marker of patients with a worse prognosis? Recently published data from the ESCAPE registry may be informative.[33] The ESCAPE registry enrolled 439 patients excluded from the ESCAPE trial for not meeting the enrollment criteria, and followed them prospectively. Based on the enrolling physician perception, registry patients were classified into three major categories: "perceived to be too sick," "perceived to be too well," and "unknown." The registry patients, in general, were different in their baseline characteristics compared with the trial patients. Hypotension, advanced renal failure, higher usage of intravenous vasoactive medications, and less use of neurohormonal modification therapies (eg, ACE inhibitors, beta blockers) were more common in registry patients. The use of intravenous inotropic agents was twice as high in the registry patients and considered the hallmark of those perceived to be "too sick" to be enrolled in the trial. Registry patients were considered to be less congested, but more underperfused than the trial patients, as assessed by the enrolling physicians. However, PAC-derived data revealed a similar overall central hemodynamic profile between the trial and registry patients.

In comparison with the trial patients, registry patients had longer hospitalizations (13 vs 6 days, P<.001) and a higher 6-month mortality (34% vs 20%, P<.001). Interestingly, the outcome of registry patients who were classified as "too well to enroll" was not better than that of other subgroups. In fact, there were no statistical differences between the "too well to enroll" and the "too sick to enroll" subgroups respectively in length of stay (11 days vs 14 days, P = .07) and 6-month mortality (39% vs 33%, P = .43). This may be because the perception of "too well" was modified by overlooked, important comorbidities.

Analyzing information from the registry database provides us with some insight into the complexity of the ESCAPE trial itself. It is obvious that the ESCAPE trial enrolled patients with lower disease severity and a better prognostic profile than the registry; this fact is confirmed by the considerably higher mortality and longer hospitalizations seen among the registry patients. Another interesting consideration is that the decision of using the PAC itself may have actually singled out patients with high-risk profiles and less favorable outcomes despite similarities in baseline hemodynamics between the trial and the registry patients. Whether PAC use in high-risk patients has an impact on their clinical outcomes now remains to be seen. In short, it is rather inappropriate to apply the results of the ESCAPE trial to higher-risk patients who require more intense approaches and a rather meticulous selection and adjustment of therapies.

Following the report of the ESCAPE trial, a large meta-analysis of 13 trials (including ESCAPE) involving 5051 critically ill patients was published by Shah and colleagues[34] Most patients (52.8%) in this meta-analysis resided in surgical care units. Because of heterogeneities in therapeutic goals and treatment options among these various trials, a random-effects model was used to compare mortality and number of days spent in the hospital among PAC and non-PAC patients. This meta-analysis showed no significant difference in mortality or days hospitalized between the two groups.

A few other trials merit commentary. The PAC-MAN is a randomized trial from the United Kingdom that investigated PAC use in the critical care setting.[8] There were 1041 patients enrolled between 2001 and 2004; 72% of them were felt to require placement of a PAC to guide vasoactive therapy. Hospital mortality, length of stay in the intensive care units, and the overall hospital length of stay were the same in the PAC and non-PAC groups. However, among the study population, only 11% were managed for heart failure symptoms. Analysis of this small heart failure subgroup showed no differences in study end points between PAC and non-PAC management.

A retrospective look at Global Utilization of Streptokinase and Tissue Plasminogen Activator for Occluded Coronary Arteries (GUSTO) II and III trials involving 26,437 patients with acute coronary syndromes was published in 2005.[35] PAC use was associated with a higher 30-day mortality in both unadjusted (OR: 8.7, 95% CI: 7.3-1.2) and adjusted (OR: 6.4, 95% CI: 5.4-7.6) analyses.

INDICATIONS FOR PULMONARY ARTERY CATHETERS IN TREATMENT OF HEART FAILURE

One must conclude from the ESCAPE trial that the PAC is no longer a standard component of the management of decompensated heart failure. The American Heart Association/American College of Cardiology (AHA/ACC) guidelines committee in its update of guidelines for management of chronic heart failure lowered the PAC indication to class II B.[36] The guideline states that PAC use might be reasonable to guide therapy in select patients with refractory end-stage heart failure (level of evidence C).

PAC use, however, should be still considered in the management of acute symptomatic heart failure when conventional treatment fails to improve the clinical condition or when volume status cannot be accurately gleaned from clinical assessment alone. PAC can be helpful when management is complicated by renal failure or persistent hypotension to ensure adequate volume status, organ perfusion, and optimal safe dosing of vasoactive drugs.

PAC can still be a useful diagnostic tool in determining the cardiac versus pulmonic etiologies of dyspnea. PAC data can generally identify cardiac origin of pulmonary edema from noncardiac causes, and distinguish between various types of hemodynamic shock when imaging modalities, laboratory data, history, and clinical examination are insufficient. The PAC provides us with the criteria needed to establish the diagnosis of pulmonary arterial hypertension and in selecting drugs, adjusting doses, and performing periodic assessment in the chronic management of the pulmonary hypertension. Finally, the PAC provides the necessary assessment of pulmonary vascular resistance and reactivity of the pulmonary vascular bed in the consideration for cardiac transplantation and/or placement of mechanical supportive devices.

A TRIBUTE TO THE PULMONARY ARTERY CATHETER

Despite the recent decline in general use, the PAC has contributed substantially to the understanding and advancement of basic cardiovascular pathophysiology and clinical cardiovascular medicine. This simple, inexpensive, easy-to-implant and relatively safe device (in experienced hands) allowed two generations of physicians to directly and serially measure central hemodynamic parameters and study the fundamentals of cardiopulmonary physiology and gas exchange in normal and provoked physiologic states (eg, pre- and postexercise), and pre- and postadministration of various cardiovasoactive drugs. PAC augmented our understanding of the hemodynamic effects of various drugs we currently use to treat a considerable number of cardiac and pulmonic diseases in humans. Categorization of drugs, such as preload-reducing and afterload-reducing agents, vasodilators, and positive or negative inotropic drugs, was largely made possible with hemodynamic data provided by PACs; and our understanding of these concepts and their therapeutic role in human disease helped us develop drugs and characterize their function. We learned from the PAC era that the overall acute hemodynamic responses to vascoactive drugs in heart failure unfortunately do not consistently or directly correspond with their long-term responses and clinical outcomes.[37–40]

Importantly, PACs made us better clinicians by allowing the simultaneous direct bedside assessment of symptoms, physical signs, findings on examination, and the central hemodynamic data and profile.

SUMMARY

The pulmonary artery catheter will likely earn a place in the history of medicine as one of the most useful tools that shaped our understanding and management of various diseases, particularly acute heart failure, decompensated chronic heart failure, and shock conditions. An intense assessment of its general application in nonacute and nonshock decompensated heart failure has now been provided by the ESCAPE trial, a landmark investigation that showed an overall neutral impact of PAC-guided therapy over therapy guided by clinical evaluation and judgment alone. The current guidelines reserve the use of PAC for the management of refractory heart failure and select conditions (eg, pulmonary hypertension, transplant evaluation). In general, the PAC remains a useful instrument in clinical situations when clinical and laboratory assessment alone is insufficient in establishing the diagnosis and pathophysiologic condition, and in guiding effective, safe therapy.

REFERENCES

1. Swan HJ, Ganz W, Forrester J, et al. Catheterization of the heart in man with use of a flow-directed balloon-tipped catheter. N Engl J Med 1970; 283(9):447–51.
2. Robin ED. Monitoring hypoxia. Int J Clin Monit Comput 1985;2(2):107–11.
3. Robin ED. A critical look at critical care. Crit Care Med 1983;11(2):144–8.
4. Robin ED. The cult of the Swan-Ganz catheter. Overuse and abuse of pulmonary flow catheters. Ann Intern Med 1985;103(3):445–9.
5. Gore JM, Goldberg RJ, Spodick DH, et al. A community-wide assessment of the use of pulmonary artery catheters in patients with acute myocardial infarction. Chest 1987;92(4):721–7.
6. Robin ED. Death by pulmonary artery flow-directed catheter. Time for a moratorium? Chest 1987;92(4): 727–31.
7. Connors AF Jr, Speroff T, Dawson NV, et al. The effectiveness of right heart catheterization in the initial care of critically ill patients. SUPPORT investigators. JAMA 1996;276(11):889–97.
8. Harvey S, Harrison DA, Singer M, et al. Assessment of the clinical effectiveness of pulmonary artery catheters in management of patients in intensive care (PAC-Man): a randomised controlled trial. Lancet 2005;366:472–7.
9. Sandham JD, Hull RD, Brant RF, et al. A randomized, controlled trial of the use of pulmonary-artery catheters in high-risk surgical patients. N Engl J Med 2003;348(1):5–14.
10. Isaacson IJ, Lowdon JD, Berry AJ, et al. The value of pulmonary artery and central venous monitoring in patients undergoing abdominal aortic reconstructive surgery: a comparative study of two selected, randomized groups. J Vasc Surg 1990; 12(6):754–60.
11. Joyce WP, Provan JL, Ameli FM, et al. The role of central haemodynamic monitoring in abdominal aortic surgery. A prospective randomised study. Eur J Vasc Surg 1990;4(6):633–6.
12. Bender JS, Smith-Meek MA, Jones CE, et al. Routine pulmonary artery catheterization does not reduce morbidity and mortality of elective vascular surgery: results of a prospective, randomized trial. Ann Surg 1997;226(3):229–36 [discussion 236–7].
13. The ESCAPE Investigators. Evaluation study of congestive heart failure and pulmonary artery catheterization effectiveness: the ESCAPE trial. JAMA 2005;294(13):1625–33.
14. Wiener RS, Welch HG. Trends in the use of the pulmonary artery catheter in the United States, 1993–2004. JAMA 2007;298(4):423–9.
15. Forssmann W. The catheterization of the right side of the heart. Klin Wochenschr 1929;45:2085–7.
16. Cournand A. Catheterization of the right auricle in man. Proc Soc Exp Biol Med 1941;46:462–6.
17. Cournand A, Bloomfield RA. Recording of right pressures in man. Proc Soc Exp Biol Med 1944;55: 34–6.
18. Cournand A, Richards DW Jr, Darling RC. Graphic tracings of respiration in study of pulmonary disease. Am Rev Tuberc 1939;40:487–516.

19. Hellems HK, Haynes FW, Dexter L. Pulmonary 'capillary' pressure in man. J Appl Phys 1949;2:24–9.

20. Connolly DC, Kirklin JW, Wood EH, et al. The relationship between pulmonary artery wedge pressure and left atrial pressure in man. Circ Res 1954;2:434–40.

21. Ganz W, Donoso R, Marcus HS, et al. A new technique for measurement of cardiac output by thermodilution in man. Am J Cardiol 1971;27(4):392–6.

22. Forrester JS, Diamond G, Chatterjee K, et al. Medical therapy of acute myocardial infarction by application of hemodynamic subsets (first of two parts). N Engl J Med 1976;295(24):1356–62.

23. Forrester JS, Diamond G, Chatterjee K, et al. Medical therapy of acute myocardial infarction by application of hemodynamic subsets (second of two parts). N Engl J Med 1976;295(25):1404–13.

24. Rao TL, Jacobs KH, El-Etr AA, et al. Reinfarction following anesthesia in patients with myocardial infarction. Anesthesiology 1983;59(6):499–505.

25. Whittemore AD, Clowes AW, Hechtman HB, et al. Aortic aneurysm repair. Reduced operative mortality associated with maintenance of optimal cardiac performance. Ann Surg 1980;192(3):414–21.

26. Berlauk JF, Abrams JH, Gilmour IJ, et al. Preoperative optimization of cardiovascular hemodynamics improves outcome in peripheral vascular surgery. A prospective, randomized clinical trial. Ann Surg 1991;214(3):289–97.

27. Rowley KM, Clubb KS, Smith GJ, et al. Right-sided infective endocarditis as a consequence of flow-directed pulmonary-artery catheterization. A clinicopathological study of 55 autopsied patients. N Engl J Med 1984;311(18):1152–6.

28. Dalen JE, Bone RC. Is it time to pull the pulmonary artery catheter? JAMA 1996;276(11):916–8.

29. Shah MR, O'Connor CM, Sopko G, et al. Evaluation study of congestive heart failure and pulmonary artery catheterization effectiveness (ESCAPE): design and rationale. Am Heart J 2001;141(4):528–35.

30. Stevenson LW, Sietsema K, Tillisch JH, et al. Exercise capacity for survivors of cardiac transplantation or sustained medical therapy for stable heart failure. Circulation 1990;81(1):78–85.

31. Stevenson LW, Brunken RC, Belil D, et al. Afterload reduction with vasodilators and diuretics decreases mitral regurgitation during upright exercise in advanced heart failure. J Am Coll Cardiol 1990;15(1):174–80.

32. Steimle AE, Stevenson LW, Chelimsky-Fallick C, et al. Sustained hemodynamic efficacy of therapy tailored to reduce filling pressures in survivors with advanced heart failure. Circulation 1997;96(4):1165–72.

33. Allen LA, Rogers JG, Warnica JW, et al. High mortality without ESCAPE: the registry of heart failure patients receiving pulmonary artery catheters without randomization. J Card Fail 2008;14(8):661–9.

34. Shah MR, Hasselblad V, Stevenson LW, et al. Impact of the pulmonary artery catheter in critically ill patients: meta-anaylsis of randomized clinical trials. JAMA 2005;294(13):1664–70.

35. Cohen MG, Kelly RV, Kong DF, et al. Pulmonary artery catheterization in acute coronary syndromes: insights from the GUSTO IIb and GUSTO III trials. Am J Med 2005;118(5):482–8.

36. Hunt SA, Abraham WT, Chin MH, et al. ACC/AHA 2005 guideline update for the diagnosis and management of chronic heart failure in the adult: a report of the American College of Cardiology/American Heart Association Task Force on practice guidelines (writing committee to update the 2001 guidelines for the evaluation and management of heart failure): developed in collaboration with the American College of Chest Physicians and the International Society for Heart and Lung Transplantation: endorsed by the Heart Rhythm Society. Circulation 2005;112(12):e154–235.

37. Desch CE, Magorien RD, Triffon DW, et al. Development of pharmacodynamic tolerance to prazosin in congestive heart failure. Am J Cardiol 1979;44(6):1178–82.

38. Packer M, Medina N, Yushak M, et al. Hemodynamic patterns of response during long-term captopril therapy for severe chronic heart failure. Circulation 1983;68(4):803–12.

39. Leier CV, Patrick TJ, Hermiller J, et al. Nifedipine in congestive heart failure: effects on resting and exercise hemodynamics and regional blood flow. Am Heart J 1984;108(6):1461–8.

40. Massie BM, Kramer BL, Topic N, et al. Lack of relationship between the short-term hemodynamic effects of captopril and subsequent clinical responses. Circulation 1984;69(6):1135–41.

Implantable Hemodynamic Monitors

José A. Tallaj, MD[a,b], Ish Singla, MD[a],
Robert C. Bourge, MD[a],*

KEYWORDS

- Congestive heart failure • Diastolic heart failure • BNP
- Implantable monitors • Hypervolemia • Chronicle IHM
- CardioMEMS

Heart failure (HF) is a major cause of morbidity and mortality throughout the world, and the incidence of HF is increasing.[1] HF was mentioned on more than 280,000 death certificates in 2005, being the primary cause of death in more than 57,000 deaths in the United States. In addition, HF accounts for more than 1 million hospital admissions each year.[2] The syndrome of HF is characterized most often by symptoms arising from volume overload and congestion, which are the most prominent symptoms leading to hospitalization.[3] Moreover, unresolved congestion often contributes to the high readmission rate in patients who have HF. The identification of congestion depends heavily on the clinical skills and judgment of the clinician and on the individual patient's characteristics. The assessment of the fluid status made by various noninvasive variables such as weight change, jugular venous distension, peripheral edema, and chest radiograph may be unreliable in predicting decompensation of chronic HF.[4-6] Newer biochemical markers such as B-type natriuretic peptide (BNP) help in the recognition of excess volume.[7] Even BNP levels may not predict congestion accurately in some patients,[8] however, especially those who have an increased body mass index, and the use of BNP currently is not practical for patients at home.[9] Right heart catheterization (RHC) is the reference standard method for assessing hemodynamic status, intracardiac filling pressures, cardiac output, and response to therapy in patients who

have advanced HF, but it provides only a snapshot of the patient at a given point in time, usually early morning, and usually in patients who have been fasting for the procedure. As learned recently from ambulatory hemodynamic monitoring, hemodynamic changes in patients who have HF are dynamic and often are not reflected adequately by a measurement made at a single point in time (**Fig. 1**). Over the past 15 years, implantable hemodynamics monitors (IHM) have been developed to provide ambulatory hemodynamic data that can be accessed remotely. The data obtained from an IHM assist in the evaluation of congestion in patients who have HF and help in the prognostication and management of these patients. There are several IHM systems under investigation, including the Chronicle IHM (Medtronic, Inc), HeartPOD (St Jude Medical), CardioMEMS Heart Sensor (CardioMEMS, Inc), and RemonCHF (Boston Scientific) devices. The Chronicle IHM currently is the one most studied in clinical applications.

THE CHRONICLE IMPLANTABLE HEMODYNAMIC MONITOR
Historical Perspective

The first implantable hemodynamic device consisted of a pulmonary artery (PA) balloon-tipped catheter connected to a small ambulatory recorder that patients carried with them for up to 48 hours.[10] This catheter, however, was not

This article originally appeared in *Heart Failure Clinics*, volume 5, number 2.

a University of Alabama at Birmingham, Birmingham, AL, USA
b Birmingham VA Medical Center, Birmingham, AL, USA
* Corresponding author. Division of Cardiovascular Disease, Department of Medicine, University of Alabama at Birmingham, 1900 University Boulevard, Birmingham, AL 35294.
E-mail address: bbourge@uab.edu

Cardiol Clin 29 (2011) 289–299
doi:10.1016/j.ccl.2011.03.002

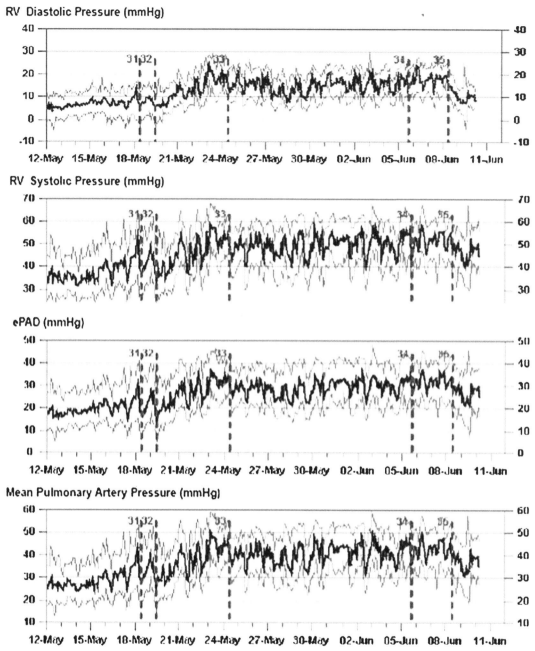

Fig. 1. Data from the Chronicle IHM in a 55-year-old woman who had dilated cardiomyopathy. Note the diurnal and day-to-day variation in the pressures and the effects of volume overload on these same pressures.

completely implantable and had to be removed after several hours to days. Development of the Chronicle implantable hemodynamic monitor system began in the early 1990s. Soon thereafter, a group in the United States and another in Europe reported the initial experience with a completely implantable hemodynamic device.[11,12] The device, which was a precursor for the Chronicle IHM, consisted of a single right ventricular (RV) lead, which had dual sensors for measuring oxygen saturation and RV pressure. These studies were small and had a relatively high incidence of lead dislodgement and other technical problems but demonstrated the feasibility of implanting a hemodynamic monitor. In the first multicenter feasibility study using this implantable device with a dual sensor in 21 patients who had HF, the oxygen sensor failed in more than half of the patients (12/21), but only two of the pressure sensors failed.[13] Given the high failure rate of the oxygen sensor, it was not included as a feature in subsequent Chronicle IHM systems.

The Chronicle Implantable Hemodynamic Monitor

The Chronicle IHM (**Fig. 2**), developed by Medtronic, Inc (Minneapolis, MN, USA) is implanted subcutaneously, similar to a pacemaker, into the pectoral region. A transvenous lead is placed in the RV outflow tract. This lead carries sensors designed to monitor heart rate, temperature, and RV systolic and diastolic pressures continuously. The change in RV pressure over time (RV dP/dt) also is measured as an index of contractility. The positive dP/dt or maximum rate of pressure is used to estimate the diastolic PA pressure (ePAD) from the RV pressure wave, which corresponds to the opening of the pulmonary valve at the end of isovolumetric contraction when the RV pressure exceeds the PA pressure. The ePAD closely approximates the left ventricular end-diastolic pressure in the absence of significant lung pathology or pulmonary arterial hypertension. Pre-ejection and systolic time intervals also can be obtained using the relationship between the RV dP/dt and the R wave of the EKG. The pre-ejection interval equals the time from the R wave to the maximal increase in RV pressure (positive RV dP/dt). The systolic time interval equals the time from the R wave to the maximal decrease in RV pressure (negative RV dP/dt).[14]

The Chronicle IHM contains a lithium–magnesium dioxide power source, integrated circuits, a motion-detection sensor, random access memory for data storage, and a radiofrequency transmission coil sealed into a titanium can. The device can store calculated mean data

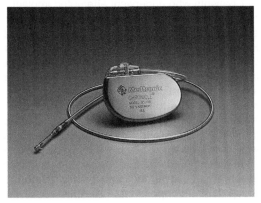

Fig. 2. Chronicle IHM system. (*Courtesy of* Medtronic, Inc, Minneapolis, MN; with permission.)

continuously over a programmable period, record real-time beat-to-beat changes in hemodynamics, and store real-time waveforms when triggered. The Chronicle data are downloaded by telephone to a central computer server via any telephone connection using a patient-used interactive remote monitor that interrogates the Chronicle device via a light-weight wand using radiofrequency transmission.[15] To correct for varying ambient atmospheric pressures, each patient wears a small external pressure reference that calibrates the IHM to changes in barometric pressure. This external device also can be used to trigger the device into a high-resolution recording mode with a reference to the triggered time recorded in the device. The Chronicle IHM data and waveforms are viewed via the Internet through the Chronicle Web site, and patient therapy is directed in accordance with the remotely acquired information. Because most patients who have systolic HF also are at risk for sudden death, the new generation of Chronicle IHM combines a pressure-sensing system for continuous hemodynamic monitoring with implantable cardioverter defibrillator (ICD) therapy designed for protection against sudden death.[16]

Clinical Experience with the Chronicle Implantable Hemodynamic Monitor

In 2002, Magalski and colleagues[17] described the performance of the Chronicle IHM in 32 patients who had HF. The data obtained from the IHM was tested against RHC, under a variety of physiologic perturbations, at 3, 6, and 12 months. There was excellent correlation between the data obtained by the Chronicle IHM and that obtained at the time of the RHC (**Fig. 3**). The correlation coefficients were 0.96 and 0.94 for RV systolic pressure, 0.96 and 0.83 for RV diastolic pressure, and 0.87 and 0.87 for ePAD at implantation and 1 year, respectively. Device- and procedure-related adverse events included one pressure sensor failure at the time of implantation, complete heart block requiring pacemaker implantation in another patient, two prolonged implantations caused by difficulties in lead calibration, one small pneumothorax, one pocket hematoma, and one incision line infection. Showing that the data obtained from the Chronicle IHM were reliable and reproducible, this study provided the framework for subsequent studies assessing the clinical utility of these devices. Subsequently, a multicenter, nonrandomized study prospectively examined the characteristics of continuously measured RV hemodynamic information from an IHM in 32 patients who had HF.[18] The measurements

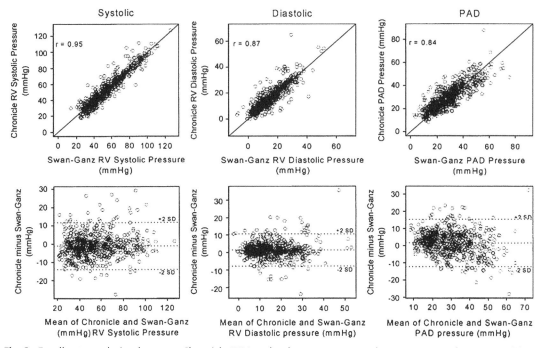

Fig. 3. Excellent correlation between Chronicle IHM and pulmonary artery catheter pressures. (*From* Magalski A, Adamson P, Gadler F, et al. Continuous ambulatory right heart pressure measurements with an implantable hemodynamic monitor: a multicenter 12-month follow-up study of patients with chronic heart failure. J Card Fail 2002;8:67; with permission.)

obtained were blinded to the physicians for the first 9 months and then were made available for the duration of the study (up to 17 months of patient follow-up). By using the data obtained by the Chronicle IHM, the hospitalization rate decreased from 1.08 per patient-year in the blind period to 0.47 per patient-year with the use of the hemodynamic data. Interestingly, during 36 volume-overload events, increases in RV systolic pressure occurred 4 ± 2 days before the event. This study was the first to suggest that a clinical benefit could be obtained by adjusting patients' therapy based on the hemodynamic data obtained from an IHM. Subsequently, 148 patients were evaluated for safety and reliability in phase I and II studies in the United States and Europe.[19] This procedure proved to be relatively easy, with very little risk of lead dislodgement (6%) and with a rate of peri-implantation events similar to those observed with the implantation of a single-chamber pacemaker system.

This initial experience paved the way for a prospective, randomized control trial, the Chronicle Offers Management to Patients with Advanced Signs and Symptoms of Heart Failure (COMPASS-HF) study.[20] This study randomly assigned 274 New York Heart Association (NYHA) class III and IV patients who had HF to either Chronicle-based

therapy or control for 6 months. All patients received optimal medical therapy, but the hemodynamic information from the monitor was used to guide patient management only in the Chronicle group. Primary end points included freedom from system-related complications, freedom from pressure-sensor failure, and reduction in the rate of HF-related events (hospitalizations and emergency or urgent care visits requiring intravenous therapy). The two safety end points were met with no pressure sensor failures, and system-related complications occurred in only 8% of the 277 patients who underwent attempted implantation (all but four complications were resolved successfully). There was a 21% reduction of all HF-related events in the Chronicle group, but this difference was not statistically significant ($P = .33$) (**Fig. 4**A). A retrospective analysis showed a statistically significant 36% improvement in the time to reduction of the time to first hospitalization for HF in the Chronicle group ($P = .03$) (**Fig. 4**B). It is possible that the study was underpowered to show a significant difference between groups, because the expected event rate was lower than expected in the control group (0.86 as opposed to the expected 1.2 per 6 patient-months), possibly related to the intensive scrutiny and contact between patients and

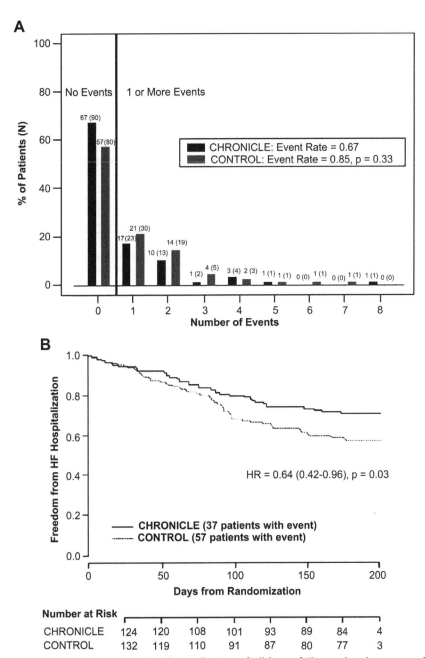

Fig. 4. Results from the COMPASS-HF trial. (*A*) Distribution of all heart failure–related events and (*B*) Kaplan-Meier curves of survival free from a heart failure–related hospitalization.

clinic/research personnel. In addition, as noted in **Table 1**, the effect of Chronicle-guided care was consistent in all but one subgroup, the NYHA classification.[21] There were more events in NYHA class IV patients in the Chronicle group than in the control group. In retrospect, the class IV patients randomly assigned to the Chronicle group were sicker, with significantly higher creatinine levels and lower scores for distance walked in

6 minutes.[22] An ongoing trial, REDUCing Events in Patients with chronic Heart Failure (REDUCEhf), is evaluating the effect of the Chronicle ICD, a dual ICD and IHM, in reducing HF-related events and mortality.

The ability of the Chronicle IHM system to estimate flow, and therefore cardiac output, was evaluated recently in a group of patients who had PA hypertension. Estimated cardiac output

Table 1
Results of the COMPASS-HF per prespecified group

Subgroup (% Patients)	Events in Chronicle Group	Events in Control Group	Interaction P-Value (Poisson Negative Binomial)	
Systolic HF (74%)	65	88	0.95	0.95
Diastolic HF (26%)	19	25		
Ischemic (46%)	46	25	0.95	0.86
Non-ischemic (54%)	38	60		
NYHA Class III (85%)	58	99	0.01	0.08
NYHA Class IV (15%)	26	14		
No device used (60%)	37	64	0.15	0.31
Device used (40%)	47	49		

Note that all groups are similar except for NYHA class.
Data from Bourge RC. The Chronicle Offers Management to Patients with Advanced Signs and Symptoms of heart failure (COMPASS-HF) study. Late-breaking trials II. Presented at American College of Cardiology Annual Scientific Sessions. Orlando (FL), March 8, 2005.

was based on RV pressure waveforms, which had excellent correlation to that measured by Fick cardiac output measurements.[23] The intermediate long-term accuracy of these estimates are not yet known.

Clinical Applications and Examples

The Chronicle IHM has become a powerful teaching and investigational tool for the centers familiar with it use. In addition to monitoring pressure and volume status, it has been used to diagnose sleep apnea and exercise intolerance and even to expose those patients who presumably are compliant with the recommended exercise program but for whom the Chronicle IHM activity monitor never changes. In addition, the Chronicle IHM has been used to optimize the settings of biventricular pacemaker[24] to manage volume status in dialysis patients who have left ventricular dysfunction[25] and in patients who have pulmonary arterial hypertension.

The following examples describe a few cases of patient management.

Example # 1

A transplant evaluation was triggered in a 55-year-old woman who had volume overload and renal insufficiency (**Fig. 5**), the patient pictured in **Fig. 1**, with widely fluctuating hemodynamics requiring repeated additional diuretic doses. An RHC performed per protocol as part of the evaluation for transplantation showed adequate hemodynamics (pulmonary capillary wedge pressure, 18–20 mm Hg; PA pressure, 40/18 mm Hg; right atrial pressure 10 mm Hg; all with preserved cardiac output). The patient called back 2 days

later, again volume overloaded and short of breath. As noted from a review of the hemodynamic data obtained from the Chronicle IHM, the RHC was done when the patient showed the best hemodynamic profile seen in months (see the solid arrow in **Fig. 5**). This improvement might have resulted in part from her fasting that morning (other than medication) or from better compliance with salt restriction and medications in the day or 2 before the catheterization. As seen, significant deterioration in hemodynamics started hours after the catheterization procedure, requiring hospitalization for parenteral therapy.

Example # 2

A 50-year-old woman who had severe diastolic dysfunction from hypertrophic cardiomyopathy underwent an exercise treadmill test (**Fig. 6**). At baseline the Chronicle IHM showed pressures in the optivolemic range. As soon as exercise began, and before stage I of a regular Bruce protocol was completed, the RV systolic pressure had gone from the low mid-40s to almost 100 mm Hg, and the patient became markedly dyspneic and presyncopal. These pressures returned to baseline levels within 3 minutes of recovery. This example, again, shows how dynamic intracardiac pressures can be, even in patients who have relatively normal or low pressures at rest.

THE HEARTPOD SYSTEM

The HeartPOD heart failure management system (St Jude Medical, St Paul, Minnesota) is another IHM system. It is a stand-alone left atrial pressure monitor that consists of a sensor lead implanted in left atrium via a transseptal approach, an external

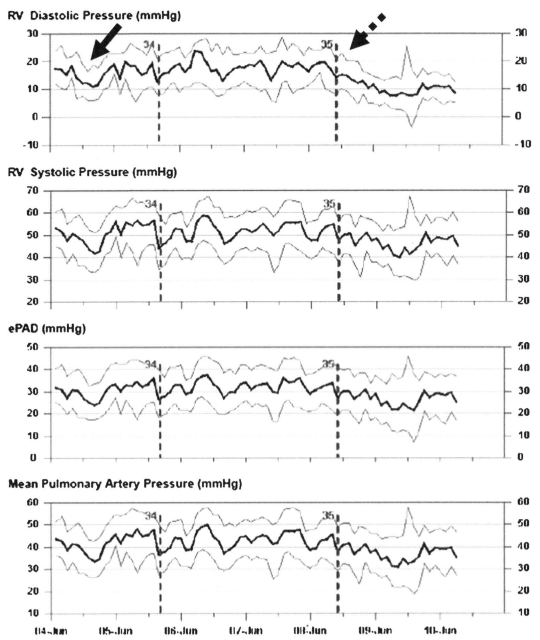

Fig. 5. Chronicle IHM hemodynamic trends from the patient in **Fig. 1**. A right heart catheterization was done as part of a transplant evaluation, with acceptable hemodynamics (*solid arrow*). Days later, however, the patient experienced symptoms of heart failure congestion (*dashed line 34*) that did not respond to oral diuretics and resulted in hospitalization for parenteral diuretics (*dashed line 35* and *dashed arrows*). Note the decrease in pressures within 24 hours of admission.

patient advisory module, and an electronic software system.[26] The sensor lead is enclosed in titanium and contains a sensing diaphragm, microstrain gauges, and a integrated circuit that digitally samples left atrial pressure, core body temperature, and intracardiac electrogram waveforms. The sensor lead is implanted via a superior subclavian vein or inferior femoral vein approach.

Following transseptal catheterization, a folding nitinol anchor affixes the sensor lead to the septum lead. The sensor lead is attached to communication module implanted in subcutaneous pocket similar to that used for a pacemaker generator. The sensor module is interrogated with a modified personal digital assistant called a "patient advisory module." During the first 6 months after

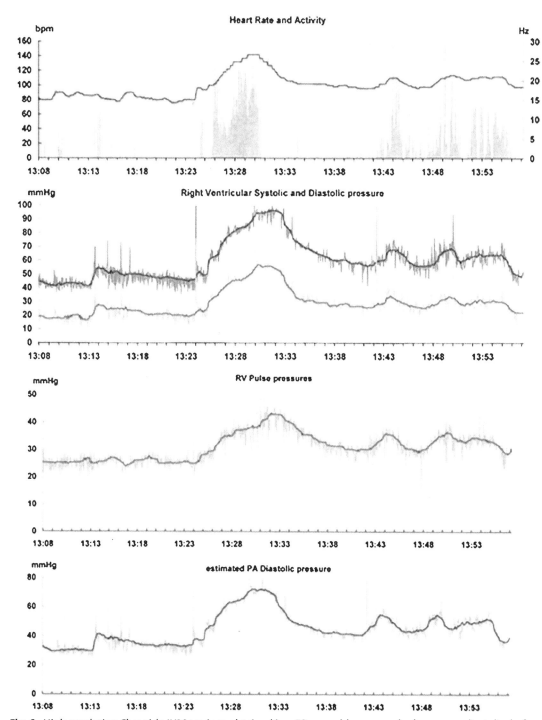

Fig. 6. High-resolution Chronicle IHM tracings obtained in a 50-year-old woman who has severe diastolic dysfunction. With minimal exercise, a significant increase in the overall intracardiac pressure is noted.

implantation patients receive aspirin and clopidogrel to prevent thrombus formation at the implant site. The information obtained from the physiologic waveforms of the patient advisory module is used as input to an individualized treatment algorithm.

The clinical feasibility of the HeartPOD system is being evaluated in the Hemodynamically Guided Home Self-Therapy in Severe Heart Failure Patients trial. The preliminary results of the first 40 patients reveal that it is safe, with a 100%

implantation success rate and with no device failures at 12 months. One disadvantage is the need for a transeptal catheterization, with its associated risks, and the relatively limited physician expertise compared with other technologies. One advantage is that the device measures left atrial pressure directly, not a surrogate for left atrial pressure (eg, PA end-diastolic pressure) as with the other devices. The clinical importance of this difference in approach is unknown.

THE CARDIOMEMS HEART SENSOR

The CardioMEMS HF Sensor Pressure Measurement System (**Fig. 7**) uses wireless technology to measure PA pressure in patients who have HF. It requires the permanent placement of a miniature pressure sensor in a distal branch of a PA. The procedure is done percutaneously through a femoral vein, with minimal risk to the patient. The HF sensor is very small, oval shaped, with rounded edges. It is composed of ultraminiaturized electrical components encased in a fused silica housing that then is encapsulated in medical-grade silicon. A change in local pressure results in a change in the electrical behavior of the components enclosed inside the housing. The coil allows electromagnetic coupling to the sensor, allowing wireless communication with the sensor without a battery or any other source of energy. Therefore it is possible to measure changes in pressure by interrogating the sensor remotely.[27] Advantages of the CardioMEMS system are the ease and (to date) low risk of insertion and device placement, the compact design, and sensor electronics. A possible disadvantage is the inability of the device, in its current iteration, to store continuous data; therefore data collection is limited to intermittent acquisition.

A recent study evaluated the accuracy of these sensor measurement systems in 12 patients who had NYHA class II to IV disease when compared with invasively measured pressures at implantation and 60 days. The CardioMEMS pressure sensor exhibited an excellent correlation with invasively measured systolic, diastolic, and mean PA pressures ($r^2 = 0.88$–0.96 at times measured).[28] Currently, a prospective, multicenter, randomized, single-blind clinical trial evaluating the safety and efficacy of the CardioMEMS pressure sensor in reducing HF-related hospitalizations is underway. Another potential advantage of this technology is that it also provides an estimate of cardiac output extracted from the PA pressure waveform. The accuracy of this approach has not been validated adequately over time and is not being used as part of the clinical management of the hemodynamic parameters in the ongoing trial.

THE REMONCHF SYSTEM

Another IHM system that uses a similar placement but different technology is the RemonCHF system (Boston Scientific, Natick, Massachusetts). This device measures the absolute pressure in the PA based on invasive, on-demand, acoustic wave technology. The Remon system consists of a pressure-sensing module enclosed in titanium case implanted in the PA via catheter using a percutaneous venous approach and an external system. The pressure-sensing module consists of an ultrasonic energy exchanger, a control chip, a pressure sensor, and a miniature battery. The micro-electromechanical system pressure sensor is used to measure the absolute PA pressure. The miniature battery allows the implant to perform pressure measurements every 10 seconds. The external components include a handheld patient unit and a clinic unit. The implant can be interrogated by the patient pressing the "start examination" button on the implant or by the clinician using clinic unit. The clinic unit also can download PA pressure data recorded on patient's handheld unit. The accuracy of PA pressures has been validated by comparison with simultaneous pressure measurements using Swan-Ganz catheterization.[29] Advantages of the device are the ease of interrogation with an internal or external ultrasonic transducer and (potentially) long device functionality. As a stand-alone system, this IHM suffers from the lack of continuous data storage (as do all but the Chronicle IHM). Clinical trials of this technology and the integration of this sensor with other devices are under development.

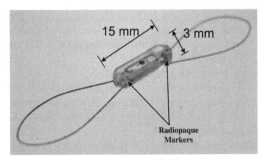

Fig. 7. The CardioMEMS heart sensor. Nitinol anchoring wires extend from the micro-electromechanical system sensor. (*Courtesy of* the Georgia Institute of Technology, Atlanta, GA; with permission.)

SUMMARY

Evaluation and management of volume status in patients who have HF is a challenge for most clinicians. In addition, such an evaluation is possible only during a personal clinician–patient interface. The ability to acquire hemodynamic data continuously with the help of implanted devices with remote monitoring capability can provide early warning of HF decompensation and thus may aid in preventing hospitalizations for HF. The data obtained also may improve the understanding of the disease process. It is important for the HF clinician to become acquainted with this type of technology and learn to interpret and use these data appropriately. With the proper use of the acquired data, morbidity and future events could be avoided with a pre-emptive adjustment of medical therapy, most often with dynamic changes in diuretics and vasodilators. There is a learning curve in managing patients with this type of technology, and mastering the learning curve is of utmost importance in demonstrating the clinical success of this kind of these devices. The monitoring function of the IHM provides data to the clinician. IHM devices, at least in terms of the data-monitoring function, do not treat the patient. Of the IHMs currently under development, the Chronicle IHM is has been best studied and has excellent reliability and long-term accuracy. Multiple ongoing studies are evaluating the safety and the efficacy of this technology in the management of patients who have HF.

One limitation of this technology is the lack of intermediate or long-term data on the accurate measurement of cardiac output (or an index of cardiac output), another important tool in the management of difficult and complicated patients and patients who have PA hypertension. Moreover, acute changes in cardiac output may be missed if the cardiac output is only measured by the arterial–venous oxygen extraction.

REFERENCES

1. Rosamond W, Flegal K, Furie K, et al. Heart disease and stroke statistics—2008 update. Circulation 2008;117:e25–146.
2. National Center for Health Statistics. Centers for disease control and prevention. Compressed mortality file: underlying cause of death. 1979-2004. Atlanta (GA): Centers for Disease Control and Prevention. Available at: http://wonder.cdc.gov/mortSQL.html. Accessed April 14, 2008.
3. ADHERE—Acute Decompensated Heart Failure National Registry. Q1 2004 National benchmark report. Atlanta (GA): Adair-Greene Healthcare Communications; 2004. p. 1–21.
4. Chakko S, Woska D, Martinez H, et al. Clinical, radiographic,and hemodynamic correlations in chronic congestive heart failure: conflicting results may lead to inappropriate care. Am J Med 1991;90:353–9.
5. Stevenson LW, Perloff JK. The limited reliability of physical signs for estimating hemodynamics in chronic heart failure. JAMA 1989;261:884–8.
6. Badgett RG, Morrow CD, Raminez G, et al. How well can the chest radiograph diagnose left sided heart failure in adults? J Gen Intern Med 1996;11:625–34.
7. Maisel AM, Krishaswamy P, Nowak R, et al. Rapid measurement of B-type natriuretic peptide in the emergency diagnosis of heart failure. N Engl J Med 2002;347:161–7.
8. Packer M. Should B-type natriuretic peptide be measured routinely to guide the diagnosis and management of chronic heart failure? Circulation 2003;108:2950–3.
9. Horwich TB, Hamilton MA, Fonarow GC. B-type natriuretic peptide levels in obese patients with advanced heart failure. J Am Coll Cardiol 2006;47: 85–90.
10. Gibbs JSR, MacLachlan D, Foc KM. A new system of ambulatory pulmonary artery pressure recording. Br Heart J 1992;68:230–5.
11. Steinhaus DM, Lemery R, Brenahan DR, et al. Initial experience with an implantable hemodynamic monitor. Circulation 1996;93:745–52.
12. Ohlsson A, Bennett T, Ottenhoff F, et al. Long term recording of cardiac output via an implantable hemodynamic monitoring device. Eur Heart J 1996;17:1902–10.
13. Ohlsson A, Kubo SH, Stainhaus D, et al. Continuous ambulatory monitoring of absolute right ventricular pressure and mixed venous oxygen saturation in patients with heart failure using an implantable hemodynamic monitor: one year multi-center feasibility study. Eur Heart J 2001;22(11):942–54.
14. Pamboukian SV, Smallfield MC, Bourge RC. Implantable hemodynamic monitoring devices in heart failure. Curr Cardiol Rep 2006;8(3):187–90.
15. Kjellström B, Igel D, Abraham J, et al. Trans-telephonic monitoring of continuous haemodynamic measurements in heart failure patients. J Telemed Telecare 2005;11(5):240–4.
16. Adamson PB, Conti JB, Smith AL, et al. Reducing events in patients with chronic heart failure (REDUC-Ehf) study design: continuous hemodynamic monitoring with an implantable defibrillator. Clin Cardiol 2007;30(11):567–75.
17. Magalski A, Adamson P, Gadler F, et al. Continuous ambulatory right heart pressure measurements with an implantable hemodynamic monitor: a multicenter 12-month follow-up study of patients with chronic heart failure. J Card Fail 2002;8:63–70.

18. Adamson PB, Magalski A, Braunschweig F, et al. Ongoing right ventricular hemodynamics in heart failure—clinical value of measurements derived from an implantable monitoring system. J Am Coll Cardiol 2003;41:565–71.

19. Stainhaus D, Reynolds DW, Gadler F, et al. Implant experience with an implantable hemodynamic monitor for the management of symptomatic heart failure. Pacing Clin Electrophysiol 2005;28:747–53.

20. Bourge RC, Abraham WT, Adamson PB, et al. Randomized controlled trial of an implantable continuous hemodynamic monitor in patients with advanced heart failure. The COMPASS-HF study. J Am Coll Cardiol 2008;51:1073–9.

21. Bourge RC. The Chronicle Offers Management to Patients with Advanced Signs and Symptoms of Heart Failure (COMPASS-HF) study. Late-breaking trials II. Presented at American College of Cardiology Annual Scientific Sessions. Orlando (FL), March 8, 2005.

22. Tallaj JA, Bourge RC, Aaron MF, et al. Continuous hemodynamic monitoring in the management of advanced heart failure patients. J Card Fail 2005; 11(6):380.

23. Karamanoglu M, McGoon M, Frantz RP, et al. Right ventricular pressure waveform and wave reflection analysis in patients with pulmonary arterial hypertension. Chest 2007;132:37–43.

24. Braunschweig F, Kjellström B, Gadler F, et al. Optimization of cardiac resynchronization therapy by continuous hemodynamic monitoring. J Cardiovasc Electrophysiol 2004;15(1):94–6.

25. Braunschweig F, Kjellström B, Söderhäll M, et al. Dynamic changes in right ventricular pressures during haemodialysis recorded with an implantable hemodynamic monitor. Nephrol Dial Transplant 2006;21(1):176–83.

26. Walton AS, Kum H. The HeartPOD implantable heart failure therapy system. Heart Lung Circ 2005; 14(Suppl 1):S31–3.

27. Castro PF, Concepcion R, Bourge R, et al. A wireless pressure sensor for monitoring pulmonary artery pressure in advanced heart failure: initial experience. J Heart Lung Transplant 2007;26(1): 85–8.

28. Verdejo HE, Castro PF, Concepcion R, et al. Comparison of a radiofrequency-based wireless pressure sensor to Swan-Ganz catheter and echocardiography for ambulatory assessment of pulmonary artery pressure in heart failure. J Am Coll Cardiol 2007;50(25):2375–82.

29. Rozenman Y, Swartz RS, Shah H, et al. Wireless acoustic communication with a miniature pressure sensor in the pulmonary artery for disease surveillance and therapy of patients with congestive heart failure. J Am Coll Cardiol 2007;49:784–9.

Epidemiology of Cardiorenal Syndrome

Robert J. Mentz, MD[a], Eldrin F. Lewis, MD, MPH[b],*

KEYWORDS

- Cardiorenal syndrome • Congestive heart failure
- Epidemiology • Management • End-of-life

The prevalence of symptomatic chronic heart failure (CHF) in the United States is estimated at 2% in those over 45 years of age with a lifetime risk of CHF estimated at 20%.[1,2] CHF is the leading cause of hospitalization in persons over age 65. Responsible for more than 1 million hospitalizations annually in the United States, CHF costs were approximately $37 billion in 2009.[3,4] In trying to improve the management of these complicated patients, the interactions between the heart and the kidney have become an area of considerable interest.[5] The presence of renal impairment is common in low and preserved ejection fraction (EF) as well as symptomatic and asymptomatic patients.[6,7] Renal dysfunction plays an important role in the progression of cardiovascular disease[8–10] and serves as an independent risk factor for morbidity and mortality in patients with heart failure (HF).[11,12] In end-stage renal disease patients, approximately 30% have CHF on initiation of dialysis[13] and patients commonly die from cardiovascular causes.[14] This interdependence of the heart and the kidney has been captured in Ronco and colleagues'[15] recent definition of the cardiorenal syndrome (CRS) (**Table 1**). The CRS includes acute and chronic conditions where the heart or the kidney serves as the primary failing organ with resulting dysfunction in both organs perpetuating the combined dysfunction through interrelated neurohormonal and hemodynamic mechanisms.[15] This definition encompasses multiple entities that have previously been reviewed in the literature separately (HF or

renal failure, worsening renal function [WRF], and diuretic resistance) and provides structure for addressing acute and longitudinal care.

This review discusses potential pathophysiologic mechanisms of the CRS; its epidemiology; inpatient and long-term care, including investigational therapies and mechanical fluid removal; and end-of-life and palliative care.

PATHOPHYSIOLOGY AND RISK FACTORS FOR CRS

Several recent reviews summarize current understanding of the pathophysiology of CRS.[14,16,17] These articles focus largely on renal insufficiency secondary to HF (CRS types I and II). Briefly, a decrease in systolic or diastolic cardiac function results in hemodynamic derangements, including low cardiac output and arterial underfilling, which are initially compensated by mechanisms of sodium retention and vasoconstriction (eg, renin-angiotensin-aldosterone system [RAAS], sympathetic nervous system, tubuloglomerular feedback [TGF], endothelin, and vasopressin) balanced with activation of vasodilatory (eg, nitric oxide, bradykinin, and prostaglandins), natriuretic, and cytokine systems.[14,16–18] These compensatory mechanisms become imbalanced due to blunting of reflexes (eg, atrial-renal) and unchecked control mechanisms (eg, lack of "escape" from salt-retaining effects of aldosterone nonosmotic release of arginine vasopressin [AVP], and elevated adenosine-mediated afferent arteriole vasoconstriction via

This article originally appeared in *Heart Failure Clinics*, volume 6, number 3.
[a] Department of Internal Medicine, Brigham and Women's Hospital, 75 Francis Street, Boston, MA 02115, USA
[b] Cardiovascular Division, Department of Medicine, Brigham and Women's Hospital, 75 Francis Street, Boston, MA 02115, USA
* Corresponding author.
E-mail address: eflewis@partners.org

Cardiol Clin 29 (2011) 301–314
doi:10.1016/j.ccl.2011.03.004

Table 1
Cardiorenal syndrome
Type I: acute CRS
Abrupt worsening of cardiac function (eg, acute cardiogenic shock or ADHF) leading to acute kidney injury
Type II: chronic CRS
Chronic abnormalities in cardiac function (eg, CHF) causing progressive and potentially permanent CKD
Type III: acute renocardiac syndrome
Abrupt worsening of renal function (eg, acute kidney ischemia or glomerulonephritis) causing acute cardiac disorder (eg, HF, arrhythmia, ischemia)
Type IV: chronic renocardiac syndrome
CKD (eg, chronic glomerular or interstitial disease) contributing to decreased cardiac function, cardiac hypertrophy, or increased risk of adverse cardiovascular events
Type V: secondary CRS
Systemic condition (eg, DM, sepsis) causing cardiac and renal dysfunction

Data from Jessup M, Costanzo MR. The cardiorenal syndrome: do we need a change of strategy or a change of tactics? J Am Coll Cardiol 2009;53(7):597–9; and Ronco C, Haapio M, House AA, et al. Cardiorenal syndrome. J Am Coll Cardiol 2008;52(19):1527–39.

TGF) in the setting of structural changes (eg, aldosterone-induced myocardial fibrosis and renovascular changes).[18,19] As a result, these maladaptative mechanisms promote a vicious cycle increasing preload and afterload and also causing oxidative stress, inflammation, and chronic renal hypoxia with resultant adverse effects on cardiac and renal function.[14,15,20] Elevated levels of cytokines, including tumor necrosis factor (TNF)-α, interleukin (IL)-1, and IL-6, in HF patients are associated with the progression of CRS via effects on negative inotropy, cardiac remodeling, and ischemic acute kidney injury.[14,15] Concomitant liver dysfunction may also play a prominent role because dysregulation of the hepatorenal reflex, vasoactive mediator-induced circulatory dysfunction, and decreased hepatic clearance of cytokines exacerbate renal and cardiac function.[21]

CRS cannot be explained by the traditional argument of poor forward flow or prerenal physiology with overdiuresis. WRF does not seem to be associated with reduced EF or poor forward flow as observed in retrospective studies[22,23] and database analysis,[24] or directly from hemodynamic data.[25] As demonstrated in the Evaluation Study

of Congestive Heart Failure and Pulmonary Artery Catheterization Effectiveness (ESCAPE) evaluating hemodynamics via pulmonary artery (PA) catheters in patients with acute decompensated HF (ADHF), cardiac output was not associated with baseline renal dysfunction or the development of WRF.[25] The only hemodynamic parameter associated with renal function was right atrial pressure. Renal dysfunction is more likely to result from raised renal vein pressure than hypoperfusion.[18] Renal perfusion depends on the difference between arterial and venous pressures, known as transrenal perfusion pressure. A growing body of literature supports the prominent role of venous congestion in WRF. Mullens and colleagues[26] used PA catheter data from 145 patients with ADHF to demonstrate that venous congestion is the most important hemodynamic factor driving WRF. Impaired cardiac output on admission and improvement in cardiac output after therapy had little impact on WRF in typical (ie, noncardiogenic shock) patients with ADHF. In contrast, higher admission central venous pressure (CVP) predicted WRF independent of baseline renal dysfunction and was associated with severity of WRF.[26] Elevated CVP has been shown to have adverse effects on sodium excretion (via stimulation of the RAAS) and renal hemodynamics with reduction in estimated glomerular filtration rate (eGFR) and renal blood flow, perhaps resulting in renal hypoxia.[16,17,26] The reduction in venous renal congestion by diuretics is a proposed mechanism for improvement in creatinine during ADHF management.

Recent data question the validity of concerns about diuretic use resulting in intravascular volume depletion (ie, prerenal physiology) during early ADHF management.[27] Patients admitted with ADHF commonly experience WRF early in their course when they are still volume overloaded rather than after aggressive diuresis.[27] When markedly volume overloaded, these patients are able to protect their intravascular volume by rapid redistribution from the extravascular compartment.[17] Although overdiuresis can eventually result in intravascular volume depletion with an elevation in creatinine and serum urea nitrogen (SUN), prerenal physiology likely does not play a major role in the early development of CRS.

Baseline renal insufficiency seems a strong independent risk factor for the development of WRF in systolic and diastolic HF.[6,22,23,28–31] Other risk factors include a history of hypertension (HTN)[25,28–31] and diabetes mellitus (DM).[6,25,28,30,32] Additional risk factors for WRF that have been reported in several retrospective analyses include older age,[22,32] a history of HF,[30,31] coronary artery disease or an ischemic etiology of CHF,[22,28] and pulmonary edema on chest radiograph or examination.[23,29] These risk factors along with others need to be validated in prospective randomized controlled trials. Although ESCAPE supported the risk factors of DM and HTN in the development of WRF, it did not independently link baseline renal function with an increased risk of development of WRF.[25] Nonetheless, even though there have been significant increases in HTN and DM with time, the incidence of WRF has not been observed to increase,[28] possibly due to changes in clinical practice and more judicious monitoring of renal function during treatment for ADHF. Thus, the conceptual model that simply having long-standing HTN, DM, and CHF results in poor forward flow and chronic kidney disease (CKD) and predisposes HF patients to WRF has not been proved. More likely, underlying DM, HTN, CHF, CKD, and other factors create a maladapative neurohormonal milieu on top of chronic systemic structural changes that culminate with increased risk for WRF that depends on the variable contribution of each of these factors in individual patients.

In addition to the baseline patient characteristics, treatment factors linked to WRF have been evaluated in several studies. Butler and colleagues[30] showed that angiotensin-converting enzyme (ACE) doses during hospitalization for ADHF are not independently associated with WRF. Jose and colleagues[33] used data from the Survival and Ventricular Enlargement (SAVE) trial involving 2231 patients with systolic dysfunction after myocardial infarction to show that ACE inhibitor use was not associated with the development of WRF. Thus, some clinicians tolerate a slight increase in creatinine to initiate proved RAAS inhibition due to documented morbidity and mortality benefits. Butler and colleagues[30] demonstrated that patients who developed WRF received higher doses of loop diuretics on the day before WRF. Similarly, Cowie and colleagues[23] found that patients who experienced WRF did not have larger outpatient loop diuretic doses, but they received higher max doses while in the hospital. ESCAPE demonstrated that in-hospital thiazide use but not loop diuretic dose was a risk factor for WRF.[25] Because diuretics activate the RAAS system and worsen the neurohormonal environment, it is appealing to incriminate their use in WRF. It is currently not known, however, whether or not diuretics have a causal relationship with WRF or if higher doses are a marker of more severe underlying disease characterized by greater diuretic resistance. Diuretic-free regimens with use of ultrafiltration (UF) are being studied for acute decompensated CHF patients.

The clinical observation of decreased diuretic responsiveness or diuretic resistance reveals

additional potential mechanisms of CRS. In HF patients, gut hypoperfusion and edema may necessitate intravenous diuretic administration due to decreased absorption. Furthermore, protein binding of loop diuretics results in an increased volume of distribution in hypoalbuminemic CHF patients and the organic acids present in renal failure inhibit the tubular secretion of diuretics.[17] Moreover, diuretic braking (with postdiuretic sodium retention) and chronic diuretic therapy-induced tubular cell hypertrophy result in enhanced sodium reuptake culminating in decreased responsiveness.[15,17]

In developing an approach to predict which patients are more likely to experience CRS, the authors remain confined to the largely unrevealing list of common comorbidities in HF patients: older, hypertensive diabetics with a history of HF and baseline renal insufficiency who receive more loop diuretics. More work is required to identify these patients earlier during management, which may enable more aggressive volume reduction and decreased length of stay.

THE EPIDEMIOLOGY OF CHRONIC CRS

Moderate to severe CKD (defined as eGFR <60 mL/min/1.73 m^2; stage III CKD) is present in 20% to 60% of HF outpatients and is associated with substantial morbidity and mortality (using the World Health Organization's anemia criteria of a hemoglobin level [below 13 g/dL in men and below 12 g/dL in women]). These estimates primarily are limited to type II and type IV CRS involving chronic abnormalities in cardiac or renal function causing progressive CKD and decreased cardiac function, respectively. These prevalence values are likely underestimated, especially type IV CRS, given the under-representation of elderly patients and those with moderate to severe renal dysfunction in the heterogenous HF studies. The Studies of Left Ventricular Dysfunction (SOLVD) revealed baseline prevalence of at least moderate CKD in 20.6% of patients in the prevention trial and 35.7% in the treatment trial but excluded patients with serum creatinine greater than 2 mg/dL or age over 79.[7] Moderate CKD was associated with an increase in all-cause mortality largely explained by an increased risk for pump failure.[7] Excluding patients with a serum creatinine greater than 3 mg/dL, the Candesartan in Heart Failure—Assessment of Reduction in Mortality and Morbidity (CHARM) and Digoxin Intervention Group (DIG) studies reported prevalence values of 36% and 46% for moderate CKD, respectively.[6,12] The DIG trial reported a threshold mortality effect with a steep increase in annual mortality when eGFR decreased below 50 mL/min/1.73 m[2].[12] In contrast, the CHARM study demonstrated a stepwise increase in mortality and admission risk with reducing eGFR.[6] Furthermore, CHARM revealed that eGFR is an independent predictor of mortality in patients with preserved EF.[6] Substudies from the Second Prospective Randomized Study of Ibopamine on Mortality and Efficacy (PRIME-II) indicated that eGFR was the strongest predictor of mortality (ie, stronger than EF).[11,34] The lowest quintile of eGFR in their study (<44 mL/min/1.73 m[2]) had a nearly 3-fold risk of mortality.[11] The prevalence values for moderate CKD women and elderly blacks are 54% and 57%, respectively.[35,36] Data from specialized ambulatory CHF clinics report a prevalence of approximately 60%.[37,38] The population-based studies are thus a better indicator of the true prevalence of moderate CKD in the outpatient CHF population (reflecting a percentage of type II and IV CRS), which is likely at least 40% to 50%. Data from the Framingham Heart Study and the Rochester Epidemiology Project in Olmsted County indicate that for incident HF cases, the average eGFR was 58.2 mL/min and the average creatinine was 1.6 mg/dL, respectively,[39,40] suggestive of moderate renal insufficiency on average in the HF community.

In their meta-analysis of HF studies with greater than or equal to 1-year follow-up, Smith and colleagues[41] report that the mortality rate was 51% in those with moderate to severe renal impairment versus 24% in those with normal renal function. Mortality increased incrementally across the range of renal function, suggesting a dose-response relationship.[41] Specifically, there was a 15% increased mortality risk for every 0.5 mg/dL increase in creatinine or a 7% increased risk for every 10 mL/min decrease in eGFR.[41] Similarly, data from the Acute Decompensated Heart Failure National Registry (ADHERE) revealed increased in-hospital mortality and length of stay with increasing stage of CKD.[24] Normal renal function was associated with an in-hospital mortality of 1.9% and length of stay of 5.3 days versus 7.6% and 7 days in stage IV kidney disease. Also, more severe kidney dysfunction was associated with increased mechanical ventilation, more frequent ICU admission and a greater incidence of cardiopulmonary resuscitation.[24] Thus, baseline renal insufficiency represents one of the strongest predictors of morbidity and mortality in HF patients with low and preserved EF.

THE EPIDEMIOLOGY OF ACUTE CRS

In trying to capture the prevalence of CRS in hospitalized patients, previous reports focused on renal dysfunction on admission for HF and WRF, which largely reflect type I and III CRS. This eliminated inpatient changes that may influence renal function, such as contrast exposure, overdiuresis, or dynamic changes in renal perfusion due to vasoactive medicines or transient low-flow states. The ADHERE registry revealed that 63.6% of ADHF patients had at least moderate renal insufficiency on admission.[24] The mean admission creatinine has increased over time from 1.46 mg/dL in 1987 to 1.62 mg/dL in 2002.[28] This increase in creatinine corresponds to a decrease in eGFR (from 73 mL/min/1.73 m[2] to 55 mL/min/1.73 m[2]) consistent with stage III CKD. With the use of advanced medical therapy and defibrillators decreasing sudden cardiac death, future admissions may involve a significantly larger population of elderly adults and those with advanced CHF and likely higher admission creatinine.

During inpatient hospitalization, WRF occurs frequently and is a subset of acute CRS. Initial studies of acute CRS used various definitions of WRF.[22,23,25,29–31] A widely accepted definition is creatinine elevation greater than or equal to 0.3 mg/dL, a threshold that has maximum sensitivity and specificity for in-hospital mortality and length of stay.[27] WRF develops early in the course of ADHF hospitalization, often within the first 3 days,[30,31] with an incidence range from 20% to 30%.[22,23,29,31] These reports are now supported by the first prospective trial in ESCAPE where the incidence was 29.5%.[25] Studies show that WRF is associated with an increased length of stay of 2 days on average,[29,30] a 2-fold higher in-hospital complication rate,[31] increased hospital costs,[29] a 3-fold increase in mortality during hospitalization,[29] an increased 6-month mortality rate (43% vs 36% in those without WRF; odds ratio for mortality of 1.62 with 95% CI of 1.45–1.82)[42] and increased mortality out to 5 years.[28] By showing that an increase in creatinine of as little as 0.2 mg/dL is associated with increased 6-month mortality, Smith and colleagues[43] revealed the prognostic importance of even small increases in creatinine. WRF seems to have associations with outcome, including in patients admitted with normal creatinine, regardless of peak creatinine and discharge values.[31,43]

In addition to baseline renal insufficiency and WRF, SUN has been recently demonstrated to have prognostic significance. Fonarow and colleagues[44] used data from the ADHERE registry to show that admission SUN greater than 43 mg/dL is the best predictor of in-hospital mortality in patients with ADHF. SUN had greater predictive power than elevated serum creatinine. Klein and colleagues[45] extended the usefulness of SUN by revealing that the change in SUN during hospitalization had the most important impact on 60-day mortality. Hemodynamic changes involving activation of the RAAS and AVP-induced SUN reabsorption in the collecting duct have been postulated as mechanisms to explain the usefulness of SUN.[16]

EXPLANATIONS FOR INCREASED MORTALITY

In addition to the pathophysiologic derangement (discussed previously), many different explanations for the increase in morbidity and mortality with renal dysfunction in HF are posited in the literature. First, renal dysfunction has been shown to limit the use of medications, such as ACE inhibitors, angiotensin receptor blocker (ARBs), and β-blockers, due to concerns about exacerbating renal function or causing hyperkalemia, especially in the elderly.[19,46–48] Also, patients with renal dysfunction have greater comorbid illnesses, such as peripheral vascular disease, dyslipidemia, and anemia.[49] The anemia of CKD is associated with poor outcome.[50,51] Al-Ahmad and colleagues[50] used data from the Studies of Left Ventricular Dysfunction (SOLVD) database to show that for every decrease in hematocrit of 1%, the mortality rate increased by 2.7%. Data from large prospective trials of CKD patients (with and without HF), however, have failed to show a benefit from treating such anemia.[52,53] Renal dysfunction also leads to abnormal calcium and phosphate metabolism with secondary hyperparathyroidism, which may have a role in abnormal vascular calcifications and arterial stiffness.[54–59] Additional explanations include elevated procoagulant biomarkers (eg, hyperhomocysteinemia),[60,61] albuminuria,[62] and uremic toxins (eg, indoxyl sulfate[63]) as well as hyponatremia[64] and other electrolyte disturbances with resultant increased arrhythmia risk.[65]

ACUTE MANAGEMENT

The first steps in the management of CRS include prevention and anticipation. Avoidance of nephrotoxic agents, including iodinated contrasts, certain higher risk antibiotics, and nonsteroidal anti-inflammatory drugs, should be undertaken whenever possible.[17] Anticipation of CRS involves early estimation of GFR via the modification of diet in renal disease equation as well as consideration of other suspected risk factors (discussed previously). Nonetheless, early diagnosis of CRS is a challenge with classic markers, such as creatinine and eGFR, which may take days to become elevated. Novel biomarkers, including serum neutrophil gelatinase-associated lipocalin (NGAL), urine IL-18, and kidney injury molecule-1 (KIM-1) may allow for earlier detection of kidney injury in the future[18] because elevation may occur much earlier in the time course of kidney injury (<12 hours) in comparison with creatinine.[15]

Once diagnosis of CRS is established, early management should involve symptom control and optimization of standard HF therapy.[17] Early symptom relief includes medications, such as diuretics and morphine for congestive symptoms, and may involve procedures, such as paracentesis and thoracentesis. Patients should be sodium and fluid restricted (<1000 mL per 24 hours of free water especially if hyponatremic[20]). Accurate daily weight is critical, because body weight is an indicator while managing CRS.[20] Early optimization of blood pressure and vasodilator therapy as well as adjuvant therapies, such as digoxin and cardiac resynchronization therapy (CRT), remains key.[17]

Despite limited trial data, diuretics have long been an essential part of CHF management. Diuretic therapy may have harmful effects on the progression of CRS, including exacerbating neurohormonal activity, worsening left ventricular (LV) function, and inducing hypovolemia and electrolyte abnormalities.[16,20] Until prospective, randomized trials with adequate power are performed to evaluate their optimization in the management of CRS, reliance is on knowledge about the principles of loop diuretics. First, consider drug half-life and the lack of a smooth dose-response curve such that a threshold level is required for diuretic effect.[17] Consequently, the dose may need to be doubled until the appropriate response occurs. Although most studies to date evaluating bolus versus continuous infusion have been small crossover trials with heterogenous populations, a Cochrane review suggests that continuous infusion of loop diuretics may provide greater diuresis, a better safety profile (less tinnitus or hearing loss), and possibly shorter length of stay and lower cardiac mortality.[66] During diuresis, patients should be closely monitored for hypotension, electrolyte depletion, and arrhythmias. Combination therapy with thiazides has been shown to increase diuretic responsiveness but careful monitoring is required due to an increased risk of hyponatremia, hypokalemia, metabolic alkalosis, and dehydration.[18] There have been reports of improved diuretic responsiveness with rotation between different loop diuretics[16] and the use of salt-poor albumin infusion in an attempt to deliver more diuretic to the kidney,[20] but future randomized trial data are needed to validate these approaches.

Although ACE inhibitors and ARBs result in significant mortality reduction in CHF, their association with worsening GFR makes continuation of their use in CRS a common clinical dilemma.[18] Trials of these neurohormonal antagonists typically excluded those with baseline renal dysfunction. Of the available trial data, there have been few subgroup analyses of those with renal dysfunction. The Cooperative North Scandinavian Enalapril Survival Study (CONSENSUS) evaluating the longitudinal use of enalapril in New York Heart Association (NYHA) class IV CHF revealed a similar risk reduction in those with renal impairment compared with those without.[18] Of the scarce data available on the use of ACE inhibitors in CHF patients who experience WRF, an association between ACE inhibitor use and WRF has not been demonstrated.[30,33] Therefore, a reasonable approach is to continue ACE inhibition despite a rise in creatinine unless renal function steadily declines or hyperkalemia develops.[67]

The onset of action for spironolactone is slower than with loop diuretics and the peak effect occurs at 48 hours.[16] The risk of hyperkalemia is of great concern with their use in the setting of CRS. Recommendations are to use mineralocorticoid antagonists with caution in those with reduced eGFR and to avoid this class when eGFR falls below 30 mL/min/1.73 m^2.[67] The 2 large trials that demonstrated the reduction in mortality in CHF with mineralocorticoid antagonists also did not use natriuretic doses.[67] Future trials are required to evaluate the use of mineralocorticoid antagonists in the acute setting.

Although there is limited literature specifically evaluating the use of β-blockers in those with CRS, post hoc analyses of randomized data from Outcomes of a Prospective Trial of Intravenous Milrinone for Exacerbations of Chronic Heart Failure (OPTIME-CHF), the Carvedilol or Metoprolol European Trial (COMET), and ESCAPE as well as registry data from the Organized Program to Initiate Lifesaving Treatment in Hospitalized Patients with Heart Failure (OPTIMIZE-HF) demonstrate that β-blocker withdrawal during admission for ADHF is associated with increased mortality.[68–71] The initiation or continuation of β-blocker therapy resulted in reduced mortality and readmission when compared with no β-blocker use in eligible patients.[71] Furthermore, β-blocker withdrawal was independently associated with a greater than 2-fold increased risk of death.[71] Continuation of β-blocker therapy was well tolerated after discharge and substantially more patients were treated as outpatients as a consequence of in-hospital continuation.[71] Medication prescription at the time of discharge has been shown the strongest predictor of long-term use.[72] Recommendations are to continue

beta blockade unless patients experience hemodynamic instability. Further randomized, prospective studies are needed to determine whether or not withdrawal of β-blockers is associated with increased risk beyond that of not receiving benefit from longitudinal use.

Renal-dose dopamine should not be used routinely in CRS management. Although several early studies showed improved kidney function with increased diuresis and natriuresis,[17] the consensus among studies with rigorous methodology is that low-dose dopamine for the treatment or prevention of ARF cannot be justified.[17] Inotropic support should be guided by the underlying physiology with or without hemodynamic guidance. Nesiritide is a recombinant analog of human brain natriuretic peptide, which seems to produce vasodilation as its main effect.[17] Early nesiritide trials and a large prospective registry suggested that nesiritide was safe in short-term management of ADHF, albeit with conflicting results on its effects on renal function, natriuresis, and diuresis.[17] In 2005, a meta-analysis of randomized, double-blind, placebo-controlled trials suggested that nesiritide may have an adverse impact on renal function (presumably by way of systemic hypotension) and may increase mortality.[73] In contrast, a meta-analysis by Arora and colleagues[74] showed no increased mortality with nesiritide.[74] The studies that demonstrated negative outcomes used nesiritide at higher doses than those currently recommended. Subsequent studies have suggested that nesiritide may have renal-protective effects when used at appropriate doses in inpatient and outpatient settings.[17] The ongoing Acute Study of Clinical Effectiveness of Nesiritide in Subjects With Decompensated Heart Failure (ASCEND-HF) may answer some of the questions on the appropriate use of nesiritide in hospitalized patients with ADHF.[75] Systematic review of the use of inotropes in acute and CHF suggests a negative impact on survival except in a few patients with severe "low output failure."[20] Therefore, because inotropic therapy may have harmful effects on the progression of CRS by further augmenting neurohormonal activation,[17] future studies need to clarify any potential use outside of maintenance of blood pressure in hemodynamically unstable patients.

The investigational therapies of vasopressin and adenosine antagonists have been shown to have positive effects on fluid loss as well as symptoms and may possibly reduce key endpoints in the case of adenosine antagonists. Vasopressin antagonists block renal water resorption (via the V2 receptor in the distal tubule and collecting duct) and vasoconstriction (V1a subtype in vascular smooth muscle cells), resulting in aquaresis, increased sodium concentration, reduced peripheral resistance and mean arterial pressure, and inhibition of AVP-mediated cardiomyocyte hypertrophy.[17] The Study of Ascending Levels of Tolvaptan in Hyponatremia (SALT) 1 and 2 showed that use of 1 of these agents (tolvaptan, a V2 antagonist) can raise serum sodium levels in patients with CHF.[76] The Efficacy of Vasopressin Antagonism in Heart Failure Outcome Study with Tolvaptan (EVEREST), which studied tolvaptan in combination with standard therapy (including diuretics) demonstrated modest effects on weight and symptoms (dyspnea and edema) in the acute setting but there was no long-term benefit on major clinical outcomes, including mortality or hospitalization.[77,78] There were no differences in renal function with the addition of tolvaptan to optimal medical therapy. Although hyponatremia in HF has been shown to correlate with mortality,[64] the use of aquaretics, such as vasopressin antagonist, have thus far have not been shown to reduce mortality and are, therefore, unlikely to play a major role in future management of acute CRS.

A1 adenosine antagonists have the potential to disrupt the TGF loop (which results in afferent arteriole vasoconstriction and decreased GFR) with potential positive effects on renal function and diuretic resistance.[17] Also, they may have beneficial inotropic effects by blocking adenosine's negative inotropic effects on cardiac A1 receptors.[17] Several small studies have shown that A1 antagonists may preserve renal function during diuresis while promoting enhanced response to loop diuretics.[17] Pilot results of the Placebo-controlled Randomized Study of the Selective A$_1$ Adenosine Receptor Antagonist Rolofylline for Patients Hospitalized with Acute Heart Failure and Volume Overload to Assess Treatment Effect on Congestion and Renal Function (PROTECT) support the use of 1 of these agents in patients with ADHF and renal impairment or diuretic resistance.[79] Rolofylline resulted in more rapid weight loss and a suggestion of reduced dyspnea, WRF, and 60-day mortality or readmission for cardiovascular or renal causes.[79] The larger follow-up study, however, did not show efficacy with this agent and future research is required.

UF offers another approach to fluid removal in the setting of volume overload, diuretic resistance, and WRF. UF harnesses a transmembrane pressure gradient to filter plasma water across a semipermeable membrane.[17] The rationale for the use of UF is based on its rapidity of fluid removal, degree of sodium clearance, and avoidance of maladaptive autoregulatory responses.[80] UF has been shown to remove more sodium and less potassium than diuretics for an equivalent volume.[17] If the removal rate and plasma-refill rate are appropriately balanced, then activation of RAAS and hypotension can be avoided.[81,82] UF may also be able to clear large biologic molecules (eg, cytokines, such as TNF-α and interleukins) that have an adverse role in the pathophysiology of HF.[80] Whether or not UF prevents WRF or improves hard endpoints in patients with CRS is unclear. Initial studies were of small sample size, included highly selected patient populations, did not report the incidence of WRF, and had short follow-up and it was unclear whether or not the patients were resistant to aggressive diuretic regimens.[17] One study showed that despite large fluid removal via UF, 50% of the patients ultimately required hemodialysis (HD) and the length of stay, costs, and mortality rates were high.[83] The Ultrafiltration versus IV Diuretics for Patients Hospitalized for Acute Decompensated Congestive Heart Failure (UNLOAD) study, a larger randomized trial of UF (n = 200), demonstrated greater fluid loss and reduced length of stay and readmission with UF compared with diuresis, but no protective effect of UF on renal function was observed.[84] Moreover, the study patient population seemed more stable than typical patients with ADHF and the groups were not controlled for the total amount of volume loss.[80] Further randomized trial data are required to support the use of UF.

The use of peritoneal dialysis (PD) in the management of treatment-resistant CHF has not been studied extensively, yet small studies report significant benefits. PD has been shown to restore diuretic responsiveness, decrease pulmonary HTN, improve NYHA class and quality of life, reduce length of stay, and substantially reduce hospitalizations.[82] As presented by Krishnan and Oreopoulos,[85] PD is associated with preservation of renal function, gentle continuous ultrafiltration, hemodynamic stability, maintenance of normonatremia, better middle-molecule clearance, and perhaps less inflammation than HD. The theory of peritoneal clearance of middle molecules or myocardium-depressing substances, such as TNF-α, ANP, myocardial depressing factor, and IL-1 and IL-6,[86] is appealing but requires further investigation. Kazory and Ross[80] elegantly discuss how the mass clearance of these compounds is low, they have short half-life periods, and they can rapidly reappear. Furthermore, the nonspecific nature of clearance means that beneficial cytokines are also lost.[80] PD offers volume removal without the rapid fall in blood pressure possible with UF.[82] In comparison with HD, PD does not require vascular access or heparin.

Moreover, PD is already established as a long-term, home-based therapy and does not required complex machinery or hospital resources. Recently, use of icodextrin-containing solutions has allowed for sustained PD over longer dwell periods. The longer dwells may allow for maintenance of euvolemia in CHF patients with 1 overnight exchange.[82] Extended dwells also likely reduce peritoneal infection risks given the small number of bag changes.[82]

Registry data in ESRD patients with CHF on PD demonstrated increased mortality with PD versus HD, thereby increasing controversy over its use.[87] The data from this registry were from 1995 to 1997, when automated PD and icodextrin solutions were less available.[82] Couchoud and colleagues[88] demonstrated similar survival rates for PD and HD in a group of 3512 patients, but there was still an increased risk of mortality with PD versus HD. Increased mortality risk in patients treated with PD may be counterbalanced by overall satisfaction, independence, and better quality of life.[89,90] Randomized trials of PD are required to further investigate its role in CRS management.

LONGITUDINAL CARE

Appropriate prescription of medications known to reduce mortality in CHF remains central to longitudinal care. Physician concerns of WRF and hyperkalemia result in underuse of medications known to reduce mortality, such as ACE inhibitors, ARBs, and spironolactone.[19,46–48] In the general HF population, prehospital cardiac regimens contained an ACE inhibitor or ARB only 53% of the time, and 48% of patients were on a β-blocker.[91] After hospitalization, only 69% were prescribed an ACE inhibitor or ARB and 59% received β-blockers.[91] In ESRD patients with LV dysfunction, 72% received β-blockade, 36% ACE inhibition, and only 25.5% the combination.[92] When appropriately titrated and monitored, these medications can be safely administered to CKD patients with similar benefits to the general population.[93] One meta-analysis demonstrated that up to a 30% increase in creatinine with ACE inhibitors that stabilizes within 2 months is associated with long-term nephroprotection.[94] Data from the CONSENSUS trial support that those patients who experience a rise in creatinine after ACE initiation may be the subgroup who achieve the greatest benefit from their use.[95] Although one-third of patients with severe HF experience a substantial increase (>30%) in creatinine with initiation of ACE inhibitors, only a small fraction of patients requires discontinuation of therapy, and creatinine levels return to baseline in most patients even

without dose adjustment.[96] Severely increased creatinine that does not stabilize could point to the possibility of underlying renovascular disease, particularly in the elderly.[97] In patients with moderate or severe renal insufficiency, therapy with ACE inhibitors should be initiated at a low dose and gradually up-titrated with careful monitoring of renal function and electrolytes.[67] Dynamic changes in renal function require intensification of monitoring.

None of the large clinical trials of β-blockers in HF has reported subgroup analyses based on renal function. One observational study evaluating β-blockers in post–myocardial infarction patients with ventricular dysfunction demonstrated a similar survival benefit in patients with creatinine greater than or less than 2 mg/dL.[98] Several studies have shown that the initiation of β-blockers may lead to initial worsening of renal function but that as cardiac function improves, renal function also improves.[18] Long-term treatment with β-blockers results in significant improvements in renal function and anemia.[18] Implications for the use of β-blockers in patients with renal dysfunction include special consideration for those that are renally excreted (atenolol, nadalol, and sotalol) versus hepatically cleared (metoprolol and carvedilol).

Data on the use of aldosterone antagonists in renal insufficiency are limited. The Randomized Aldactone Evaluation Study (RALES) demonstrated a 30% mortality reduction in patients with severe HF but excluded patients with a creatinine greater than 2.5 mg/dL.[99] The risk of hyperkalemia with aldosterone antagonists requires that renal function and electrolytes be carefully monitored. Suggestions are to avoid spironolactone in patients with a GFR less than 30 mL/min/1.73 m^2 and to use them cautiously in patients with a GFR of 30 to 60 mL/min/1.73 m^2 and at doses no higher than 25 mg daily.[67]

Digitalis does not affect CHF survival but it has been shown to result in a 28% reduction in HF hospitalizations.[100] The clearance of digitalis varies linearly with GFR such that renal dysfunction may affect its safety.[67] When used in patients with renal dysfunction, the loading dose and frequency of dosing must be modified.[67] No studies have evaluated whether or not the effects of digitalis on clinical outcomes differ by renal function.

Cardiac transplantation and left ventricular assist device (LVAD) therapy have traditionally had low clinical applicability for the majority of CRS patients given their advanced age, high surgical risk, poor prognosis, and comorbidities that preclude them from consideration.[20,101]

End-organ dysfunction, such as renal insufficiency, is associated with poor outcome after LVAD implantation.[102] GFR, however, has not consistently been shown an independent predictor of outcome in multivariate models, suggesting that use of GFR alone as a contraindication to invasive therapy is not data driven.[102] LVAD therapy has demonstrated improvements in renal function even in the absence of pre-existing low-flow.[102,103] Patients with a history of at least moderate CKD who experience improvements in renal function exhibit post-LVAD survival rates comparable with those with normal preoperative renal function.[102] Concomitant CKD is a relative contraindication to LVAD placement as clinicians attempt to determine which patients experience improved renal function after implantation.[102] Patients undergoing transplantation have lower GFR compared with 20 years ago. More often, progressive renal dysfunction, however, is a sign of transition to stage 4 HF.[17] Consequently, the presence of CRS alone or in combination with other poor prognostic signs denotes a critical time to discuss end-of-life care and possibly a shift in the balance from quantity to quality of life.

END OF LIFE

Approximately 50% of HF patients die within 5 years of diagnosis.[104] Mortality is 40% to 50% per year for those with NYHA class IV symptoms.[105] Moreover, up to half of deaths from HF are sudden.[105] Survival is best predicted by the severity of disease and symptoms after treatment and not during an exacerbation.[106] Predictors of poor prognosis in CHF include renal dysfunction, liver failure, hyponatremia,[107] cardiac cachexia,[108] and an inability to be weaned off inotropes or to restore symptoms to NYHA class III despite medical optimization[101] as well as QRS widening and reduced maximal oxygen consumption, EF, heart rate, and blood pressure.[109] Kittleson and colleagues[110] demonstrated that patients unable to tolerate ACE inhibitors due to symptomatic hypotension, progressive renal dysfunction, or hyperkalemia have more severe disease and increased mortality. Furthermore, when patients are only able to tolerate extremely low doses of HF medications, the usefulness of medication continuation is unknown. Rose and colleagues[111] demonstrated that an EF less than 25%, NYHA class IV symptoms for greater than 90 days, and maximal oxygen consumption less than or equal to 12 mL/kg/min or dependence on inotropes had a 6-month mortality of approximately 50%.

As reviewed by Goodlin in 2009,[112] through the use of appropriate medications, diet management, and other interventions, symptoms of HF can be diminished but fatigue, exertional limitations, and impaired social structure often persist. Current recommendations are to provide palliative care early in the course of HF in conjunction with therapies to prolong life.[112] Several recent reviews discuss the integration of palliative care into CHF management.[106,107,112] Some of the key points discussed in these articles include early communication and decision making about therapies, devices (implantable cardioverter defibrillator and CRT-defibrillator), goals of care, and health care proxy. Depression and patients' perceived control over their condition is tightly linked to perception of symptoms.[112] Key components of a well-rounded care plan include exercise/endurance training (eg, lower extremity strengthening and inspiratory respiratory muscle training), treatment of depression/anxiety (eg, counseling, selective serotonin reuptake inhibitors, and benzodiazepines), and management of sleep-disordered breathing (ie, continuous positive airway pressure) as well as consideration of oxygen and opioids for dyspnea.[112] The prevalence of cognitive impairment in CHF complicates recognition of worsening HF status and medication adherence.[112] Longitudinal education and psychosocial and medical support in a multidisciplinary team decrease hospitalizations, increase appropriate medication use, decrease medication errors, and improve health-related quality of life.[113] Transition toward a focus on palliation does not necessarily mean cessation of HF medications. Many patients with CHF continue taking cardiac medications indefinitely due to symptom improvement.[112] For instance, ACE inhibitors improve symptoms of HF, such as dyspnea, fatigue, orthopnea, and edema.[114] Palliative care programs have been shown to improved dyspnea, anxiety, spiritual well-being, and caregiver satisfaction and result in increased rates of death at home.[115,116] The clinical challenges of CRS will likely worsen before they get better as an aging population and HF treatment successes result in a growing number of CHF patients with end-stage cardiac and renal disease.

SUMMARY

CRS is common with 40% to 50% of stable CHF outpatients and more than 60% of those with ADHF experiencing comorbid moderate renal insufficiency. Renal insufficiency is an independent risk factor for substantial morbidity and mortality in CHF patients. Because the pathophysiology and risk factors for CRS remain incompletely understood, the optimal acute and longitudinal management is plagued by uncertainty and common clinical dilemmas. Investigational therapies, such as adenosine antagonists, and methods for extracorporeal volume removal, such as UF and PD, may offer greater success for the future of CRS management. Palliative care and the use of a longitudinal multidisciplinary team should be instituted early in the course of CHF management to provide for the optimal balance of quantity and quality of life for all patients with CHF.

REFERENCES

1. Redfield MM, Jacobsen SJ, Burnett JC, et al. Burden of systolic and diastolic ventricular dysfunction in the community: appreciating the scope of the heart failure epidemic. JAMA 2003; 289(2):194–202.

2. Lloyd-Jones DM, Larson MG, Leip EP, et al. Lifetime risk for developing congestive heart failure: the Framingham Heart Study. Circulation 2002; 106(24):3068–72.

3. American Heart Association. 2009 Heart and stroke statistical update. Dallas (TX): American Heart Association; 2009.

4. Fonarow GC. The Acute Decompensated Heart Failure National Registry (ADHERE): opportunities to improve care of patients hospitalized with acute decompensated heart failure. Rev Cardiovasc Med 2003;4(Suppl 7):S21–30.

5. Evans F, Fakunding J. NHLBI Working Group: cardiorenal connections in heart failure and cardiovascular disease. 2004. Available at: http://www.nhlbi.nih.gov/meetings/workshops/cardiorenal-hf-hd.htm. Accessed January 10, 2010.

6. Hillege HL, Nitsch D, Pfeffer MA, et al. Renal function as a predictor of outcome in a broad spectrum of patients with heart failure. Circulation 2006; 113(5):671–8.

7. Dries DL, Exner DV, Domanski MJ, et al. The prognostic implications of renal insufficiency in asymptomatic and symptomatic patients with left ventricular systolic dysfunction. J Am Coll Cardiol 2000;35(3):681–9.

8. Schrier RW. Role of diminished renal function in cardiovascular mortality: marker or pathogenetic factor? J Am Coll Cardiol 2006;47(1):1–8.

9. Go AS, Chertow GM, Fan D, et al. Chronic kidney disease and the risks of death, cardiovascular events, and hospitalization. N Engl J Med 2004; 351(13):1296–305.

10. Manjunath G, Tighiouart H, Ibrahim H, et al. Level of kidney function as a risk factor for atherosclerotic cardiovascular outcomes in the community. J Am Coll Cardiol 2003;41(1):47–55.

11. Hillege HL, Girbes AR, de Kam PJ, et al. Renal function, neurohormonal activation, and survival in patients with chronic heart failure. Circulation 2000;102(2):203–10.

12. Shlipak MG, Smith GL, Rathore SS. Renal function, digoxin therapy, and heart failure outcomes: evidence from the digoxin intervention group trial. J Am Soc Nephrol 2004;15(8):2195–203.

13. Harnett JD, Foley RN, Kent GM, et al. Congestive heart failure in dialysis patients: prevalence, incidence, prognosis and risk factors. Kidney Int 1995;47(3):884–90.

14. Bongartz LG, Cramer MJ, Doevendans PA, et al. The severe cardiorenal syndrome: 'Guyton revisited'. Eur Heart J 2005;26(1):11–7.

15. Ronco C, Haapio M, House AA, et al. Cardiorenal syndrome. J Am Coll Cardiol 2008;52(19):1527–39.

16. Sarraf M, Masoumi A, Schrier RW. Cardiorenal syndrome in acute decompensated heart failure. Clin J Am Soc Nephrol 2009;4(12):2013–26.

17. Liang KV, Williams AW, Greene EL, et al. Acute decompensated heart failure and the cardiorenal syndrome. Crit Care Med 2008;36(Suppl 1):S75–88.

18. Krum H, Iyngkaran P, Lekawanvijit S. Pharmacologic management of the cardiorenal syndrome in heart failure. Curr Heart Fail Rep 2009;6(2):105–11.

19. McMurray JJ. Failure to practice evidence-based medicine: why do physicians not treat patients with heart failure with angiotensin-converting enzyme inhibitors? Eur Heart J 1998;19(Suppl L): L15–21.

20. Pokhrel N, Maharjan N, Dhakal B, et al. Cardiorenal syndrome: a literature review. Exp Clin Cardiol 2008;13(4):165–70.

21. Slack AJ, Wendon J. The liver and kidney in critically ill patients. Blood Purif 2009;28(2):124–34.

22. Weinfeld MS, Chertow GM, Stevenson LW. Aggravated renal dysfunction during intensive therapy for advanced chronic heart failure. Am Heart J 1999;138(2 Pt 1):285–90.

23. Cowie MR, Komajda M, Murray-Thomas T, et al. Prevalence and impact of worsening renal function in patients hospitalized with decompensated heart failure: results of the prospective outcomes study in heart failure (POSH). Eur Heart J 2006;27(10): 1216–22.

24. Heywood JT, Fonarow GC, Costanzo MR, et al. High prevalence of renal dysfunction and its impact on outcome in 118,465 patients hospitalized with acute decompensated heart failure: a report from the ADHERE database. J Card Fail 2007;13(6):422–30.

25. Nohria A, Hasselblad V, Stebbins A, et al. Cardiorenal interactions: insights from the ESCAPE trial. J Am Coll Cardiol 2008;51(13):1268–74.

26. Mullens W, Abrahams Z, Francis GS, et al. Importance of venous congestion for worsening of renal function in advanced decompensated heart failure. J Am Coll Cardiol 2009;53(7):589–96.

27. Gottlieb SS, Abraham W, Butler J, et al. The prognostic importance of different definitions of worsening renal function in congestive heart failure. J Card Fail 2002;8(3):136–41.

28. Owan TE, Hodge DO, Herges RM, et al. Secular trends in renal dysfunction and outcomes in hospitalized heart failure patients. J Card Fail 2006; 12(4):257–62.

29. Krumholz HM, Chen YT, Vaccarino V, et al. Correlates and impact on outcomes of worsening renal function in patients > or =65 years of age with heart failure. Am J Cardiol 2000;85(9):1110–3.

30. Butler J, Forman DE, Abraham WT, et al. Relationship between heart failure treatment and development of worsening renal function among hospitalized patients. Am Heart J 2004;147(2):331–8.

31. Forman DE, Butler J, Wang Y, et al. Incidence, predictors at admission, and impact of worsening renal function among patients hospitalized with heart failure. J Am Coll Cardiol 2004;43(1):61–7.

32. Knight EL, Glynn RJ, McIntyre KM, et al. Predictors of decreased renal function in patients with heart failure during angiotensin-converting enzyme inhibitor therapy: results from the studies of left ventricular dysfunction (SOLVD). Am Heart J 1999;138(5 Pt 1):849–55.

33. Jose P, Skali H, Anavekar N, et al. Increase in creatinine and cardiovascular risk in patients with systolic dysfunction after myocardial infarction. J Am Soc Nephrol 2006;17(10):2886–91.

34. Smilde TD, Hillege HL, Navis G, et al. Impaired renal function in patients with ischemic and nonischemic chronic heart failure: association with neurohormonal activation and survival. Am Heart J 2004;148(1):165–72.

35. Bibbins-Domingo K, Lin F, Vittinghoff E, et al. Renal insufficiency as an independent predictor of mortality among women with heart failure. J Am Coll Cardiol 2004;44(8):1593–600.

36. Smith GL, Shlipak MG, Havranek EP, et al. Race and renal impairment in heart failure: mortality in blacks versus whites. Circulation 2005;111(10): 1270–7.

37. de Silva R, Nikitin NP, Witte KK, et al. Incidence of renal dysfunction over 6 months in patients with chronic heart failure due to left ventricular systolic dysfunction: contributing factors and relationship to prognosis. Eur Heart J 2006;27(5): 569–81.

38. McAlister FA, Ezekowitz J, Tonelli M, et al. Renal insufficiency and heart failure: prognostic and therapeutic implications from a prospective cohort study. Circulation 2004;109(8):1004–9.

39. Lee DS, Gona P, Vasan RS, et al. Relation of disease pathogenesis and risk factors to heart failure with preserved or reduced ejection fraction: insights from the Framingham heart study of the national heart, lung, and blood institute. Circulation 2009;119(24):3070–7.

40. Dunlay SM, Redfield MM, Weston SA, et al. Hospitalizations after heart failure diagnosis a community perspective. J Am Coll Cardiol 2009;54(18):1695–702.

41. Smith GL, Lichtman JH, Bracken MB, et al. Renal impairment and outcomes in heart failure: systematic review and meta-analysis. J Am Coll Cardiol 2006;47(10):1987–96.

42. Damman K, Navis G, Voors AA, et al. Worsening renal function and prognosis in heart failure: systematic review and meta-analysis. J Card Fail 2007;13(8):599–608.

43. Smith GL, Vaccarino V, Kosiborod M, et al. Worsening renal function: what is a clinically meaningful change in creatinine during hospitalization with heart failure? J Card Fail 2003;9(1):13–25.

44. Fonarow GC, Adams KF Jr, Abraham WT, et al. Risk stratification for in-hospital mortality in acutely decompensated heart failure: classification and regression tree analysis. JAMA 2005; 293(5):572–80.

45. Klein L, Massie BM, Leimberger JD, et al. Admission or changes in renal function during hospitalization for worsening heart failure predict postdischarge survival: results from the Outcomes of a Prospective Trial of Intravenous Milrinone for Exacerbations of Chronic Heart Failure (OPTIME-CHF). Circ Heart Fail 2008;1(1):25–33.

46. Houghton AR, Cowley AJ. Why are angiotensin converting enzyme inhibitors underutilised in the treatment of heart failure by general practitioners? Int J Cardiol 1997;59(1):7–10.

47. Ahmed A, Allman RM, DeLong JF, et al. Age-related underutilization of angiotensin-converting enzyme inhibitors in older hospitalized heart failure patients. South Med J 2002;95(7):703–10.

48. Masoudi FA, Rathore SS, Wang Y, et al. National patterns of use and effectiveness of angiotensin-converting enzyme inhibitors in older patients with heart failure and left ventricular systolic dysfunction. Circulation 2004;110(6):724–31.

49. Al-Ahmad A, Sarnak MJ, Salem DN, et al. Cause and management of heart failure in patients with chronic renal disease. Semin Nephrol 2001;21(1): 3–12.

50. Al-Ahmad A, Rand WM, Manjunath G, et al. Reduced kidney function and anemia as risk factors for mortality in patients with left ventricular dysfunction. J Am Coll Cardiol 2001;38(4):955–62.

51. McClellan WM, Flanders WD, Langston RD, et al. Anemia and renal insufficiency are independent risk factors for death among patients with congestive heart failure admitted to community hospitals: a population-based study. J Am Soc Nephrol 2002;13(7):1928–36.

52. Singh AK, Szczech L, Tang KL, et al. Correction of anemia with epoetin alfa in chronic kidney disease. N Engl J Med 2006;355:2085–98.

53. Drueke TB, Locatelli F, Clyne N, et al. Normalization of hemoglobin level in patients with chronic kidney disease and anemia. N Engl J Med 2006;355: 2071–84.

54. Goodman WG, Goldin J, Kuizon BD, et al. Coronary-artery calcification in young adults with end-stage renal disease who are undergoing dialysis. N Engl J Med 2000;342(20):1478–83.

55. Block GA, Port FK. Re-evaluation of risks associated with hyperphosphatemia and hyperparathyroidism in dialysis patients: recommendations for a change in management. Am J Kidney Dis 2000; 35(6):1226–37.

56. Sadeghi HM, Stone GW, Grines CL, et al. Impact of renal insufficiency in patients undergoing primary angioplasty for acute myocardial infarction. Circulation 2003;108(22):2769–75.

57. Russo D, Palmiero G, De Blasio AP, et al. Coronary artery calcification in patients with CRF not undergoing dialysis. Am J Kidney Dis 2004;44:1024–30.

58. Ketteler M, Schlieper G, Floege J. Calcification and cardiovascular health: new insights into an old phenomenon. Hypertension 2006;47:1027–34.

59. Schiffrin EL, Lipman ML, Mann JF. Chronic kidney disease: effects on the cardiovascular system. Circulation 2007;116:85–97.

60. Shlipak MG, Fried LF, Crump C, et al. Elevations of inflammatory and procoagulant biomarkers in elderly persons with renal insufficiency. Circulation 2003;107(1):87–92.

61. Boushey CJ, Beresford SA, Omenn GS, et al. A quantitative assessment of plasma homocysteine as a risk factor for vascular disease. Probable benefits of increasing folic acid intakes. JAMA 1995;274(13):1049–57.

62. Gerstein HC, Mann JF, Yi Q, et al. Albuminuria and risk of cardiovascular events, death, and heart failure in diabetic and nondiabetic individuals. JAMA 2001;286(4):421–6.

63. Taki K, Tsuruta Y, Niwa T. Indoxyl sulfate and atherosclerotic risk factors in hemodialysis patients. Am J Nephrol 2007;27(1):30–5.

64. Lee WH, Packer M. Prognostic importance of serum sodium concentration and its modification by converting-enzyme inhibition in patients with severe chronic heart failure. Circulation 1986; 73(2):257–67.

65. Leier CV, Dei Cas L, Metra M. Clinical relevance and management of the major electrolyte abnormalities in congestive heart failure: hyponatremia, hypokalemia, and hypomagnesemia. Am Heart J 1994;128(3):564–74.

66. Salvador DR, Rey NR, Ramos GC, et al. Continuous infusion versus bolus injection of loop diuretics in congestive heart failure. Cochrane Database Syst Rev 2005;3:CD003178.

67. Shlipak MG. Pharmacotherapy for heart failure in patients with renal insufficiency. Ann Intern Med 2003;138(11):917–24.

68. Gattis WA, O'Connor CM, Leimberger JD, et al. Clinical outcomes in patients on beta-blocker therapy admitted with worsening chronic heart failure. Am J Cardiol 2003;91(2):169–74 OPTIME.

69. Metra M, Torp-Pedersen C, Cleland JG, et al. Should beta-blocker therapy be reduced or withdrawn after an episode of decompensated heart failure? Results from COMET. Eur J Heart Fail 2007;9(9):901–9.

70. Butler J, Young JB, Abraham WT, et al. Beta-blocker use and outcomes among hospitalized heart failure patients. J Am Coll Cardiol 2006;47(12):2462–9.

71. Fonarow GC, Abraham WT, Albert NM, et al. Influence of beta-blocker continuation or withdrawal on outcomes in patients hospitalized with heart failure: findings from the OPTIMIZE-HF program. J Am Coll Cardiol 2008;52(3):190–9.

72. Butler J, Arbogast PG, BeLue R, et al. Outpatient adherence to beta-blocker therapy after acute myocardial infarction. J Am Coll Cardiol 2002; 40(9):1589–95.

73. Sackner-Bernstein JD, Skopicki HA, Aaronson KD. Risk of worsening renal function with nesiritide in patients with acutely decompensated heart failure. Circulation 2005;111(12):1487–91.

74. Arora RR, Venkatesh PK, Molnar J. Short and long-term mortality with nesiritide. Am Heart J 2006; 152(6):1084–90.

75. ASCEND-HF. Double-blind, placebo-controlled, multicenter acute study of clinical effectiveness of nesiritide in subjects with decompensated heart failure. Available at: http://clinicaltrials.gov/ct2/show/NCT00475852. Accessed January 10, 2010.

76. Schrier RW, Gross P, Gheorghiade M, et al. Tolvaptan, a selective oral vasopressin V2-receptor antagonist, for hyponatremia. N Engl J Med 2006; 355(20):2099–112.

77. Gheorghiade M, Niazi I, Ouyang J, et al. Vasopressin V2-receptor blockade with tolvaptan in patients with chronic heart failure: results from a double-blind, randomized trial. Circulation 2003; 107(21):2690–6.

78. Gheorghiade M, Gattis WA, O'Connor CM, et al. Effects of tolvaptan, a vasopressin antagonist, in patients hospitalized with worsening heart failure: a randomized controlled trial. JAMA 2004; 291(16):1963–71.

79. Cotter G, Dittrich HC, Weatherley BD, et al. The PROTECT pilot study: a randomized, placebo-controlled, dose-finding study of the adenosine A1 receptor antagonist rolofylline in patients with

acute heart failure and renal impairment. J Card Fail 2008;14(8):631–40.

80. Kazory A, Ross EA. Contemporary trends in the pharmacological and extracorporeal management of heart failure: a nephrologic perspective. Circulation 2008;117(7):975–83.

81. Jessup M, Costanzo MR. The cardiorenal syndrome: do we need a change of strategy or a change of tactics? J Am Coll Cardiol 2009;53(7):597–9.

82. Khalifeh N, Vychytil A, Hörl WH. The role of peritoneal dialysis in the management of treatment-resistant congestive heart failure: a European perspective. Kidney Int Suppl 2006;103:S72–5.

83. Liang KV, Hiniker AR, Williams AW, et al. Use of a novel ultrafiltration device as a treatment strategy for diuretic resistant, refractory heart failure: initial clinical experience in a single center. J Card Fail 2006;12(9):707–14.

84. Costanzo MR, Guglin ME, Saltzberg MT, et al. Ultrafiltration versus intravenous diuretics for patients hospitalized for acute decompensated heart failure. J Am Coll Cardiol 2007;49(6):675–83.

85. Krishnan A, Oreopoulos DG. Peritoneal dialysis in congestive heart failure. Adv Perit Dial 2007;23:82–9.

86. Gotloib L, Fudin R, Yakubovich M, et al. Peritoneal dialysis in refractory end-stage congestive heart failure: a challenge facing a no-win situation. Nephrol Dial Transplant 2005;20(Suppl 7):vii32–6.

87. Stack AG, Molony DA, Rahman NS, et al. Impact of dialysis modality on survival of new ESRD patients with congestive heart failure in the United States. Kidney Int 2003;64(3):1071–9.

88. Couchoud C, Stengel B, Landais P, et al. The renal epidemiology and information network (REIN): a new registry for end-stage renal disease in France. Nephrol Dial Transplant 2006;21:411–8.

89. Kirchgessner J, Pera-Chang M, Klinkner G, et al. Satisfaction with care in peritoneal dialysis patients. Kidney Int 2006;70:1325–31.

90. Frimat L, Durand PY, Loos-Avay C, et al. Impact of first dialysis modality on outcome of patients contraindicated for kidney transplant. Perit Dial Int 2006;26:231–9.

91. Gheorghiade M, Filippatos G. Reassessing treatment of acute heart failure syndromes: the ADHERE registry. Eur Heart J 2005;7(Suppl B):B13–9.

92. Roy P, Bouchard J, Amyot R, et al. Prescription patterns of pharmacological agents for left ventricular systolic dysfunction among hemodialysis patients. Am J Kidney Dis 2006;48(4):645–51.

93. Ruggenenti P, Perna A, Remuzzi G. ACE inhibitors to prevent end-stage renal disease: when to start and why possibly never to stop: a post hoc analysis of the REIN trial results. Ramipril efficacy in nephropathy. J Am Soc Nephrol 2001;12(12):2832–7.

94. Bakris GL, Weir MR. Angiotensin-converting enzyme inhibitorassociated elevations in serum creatinine: is this a cause for concern? Arch Intern Med 2000;160:685–93.

95. Effects of enalapril on mortality in severe congestive heart failure. Results of the Cooperative North Scandinavian Enalapril Survival Study (CONSENSUS). The CONSENSUS Trial Study Group. N Engl J Med 1987;316(23):1429–35.

96. Ljungman S, Kjekshus J, Swedberg K. Renal function in severe congestive heart failure during treatment with enalapril (the Cooperative North Scandinavian Enalapril Survival Study [CONSENSUS] Trial). Am J Cardiol 1992;70(4):479–87.

97. MacDowall P, Kalra PA, O'Donoghue DJ, et al. Risk of morbidity from renovascular disease in elderly patients with congestive cardiac failure. Lancet 1998;352(9121):13–6.

98. Shlipak MG, Browner WS, Noguchi H, et al. Comparison of the effects of angiotensin converting-enzyme inhibitors and beta blockers on survival in elderly patients with reduced left ventricular function after myocardial infarction. Am J Med 2001;110(6):425–33.

99. Pitt B, Zannad F, Remme WJ, et al. The effect of spironolactone on morbidity and mortality in patients with severe heart failure. Randomized Aldactone Evaluation Study Investigators. N Engl J Med 1999;341(10):709–17.

100. The effect of digoxin on mortality and morbidity in patients with heart failure. The Digitalis Investigation Group. N Engl J Med 1997;336(8):525–33.

101. Wilson SR, Mudge GH Jr, Stewart GC, et al. Evaluation for a ventricular assist device: selecting the appropriate candidate. Circulation 2009;119(16):2225–32.

102. Sandner SE, Zimpfer D, Zrunek P, et al. Renal function and outcome after continuous flow left ventricular assist device implantation. Ann Thorac Surg 2009;87(4):1072–8.

103. Kamdar F, Boyle A, Liao K, et al. Effects of centrifugal, axial, and pulsatile left ventricular assist device support on end-organ function in heart failure patients. J Heart Lung Transplant 2009;28(4):352–9.

104. Heart disease and stroke statistics—2004 update. Dallas (TX): American Heart Association; 2000.

105. Stevenson WG, Stevenson LW. Prevention of sudden death in heart failure. J Cardiovasc Electrophysiol 2001;12(1):112–4.

106. Pantilat SZ, Steimle AE. Palliative care for patients with heart failure. JAMA 2004;291(20):2476–82.

107. Hauptman PJ, Havranek EP. Integrating palliative care into heart failure care. Arch Intern Med 2005;165(4):374–8.

108. Anker SD, Chua TP, Ponikowski P, et al. Hormonal changes and catabolic/anabolic imbalance in chronic heart failure and their importance for cardiac cachexia. Circulation 1997;96(2):526–34.

109. Aaronson KD, Schwartz JS, Chen TM, et al. Development and prospective validation of a clinical index to predict survival in ambulatory patients referred for cardiac transplant evaluation. Circulation 1997;95(12):2660–7.

110. Kittleson M, Hurwitz S, Shah MR, et al. Development of circulatory-renal limitations to angiotensin-converting enzyme inhibitors identifies patients with severe heart failure and early mortality. J Am Coll Cardiol 2003;41(11):2029–35.

111. Rose EA, Gelijns AC, Moskowitz AJ, et al. Long-term mechanical left ventricular assistance for end-stage heart failure. N Engl J Med 2001; 345(20):1435–43.

112. Goodlin SJ. Palliative care in congestive heart failure. J Am Coll Cardiol 2009;54(5):386–96.

113. Phillips CO, Wright SM, Kern DE, et al. Comprehensive discharge planning with postdischarge support for older patients with congestive heart failure: a meta-analysis. JAMA 2004;291(11):1358–67.

114. A placebo-controlled trial of captopril in refractory chronic congestive heart failure. Captopril Multicenter Research Group. J Am Coll Cardiol 1983; 2(4):755–63.

115. Rabow MW, Dibble SL, Pantilat SZ, et al. The comprehensive care team: a controlled trial of outpatient palliative medicine consultation. Arch Intern Med 2004;164(1):83–91.

116. Brumley R, Enguidanos S, Jamison P, et al. Increased satisfaction with care and lower costs: results of a randomized trial of in-home palliative care. J Am Geriatr Soc 2007;55(7):993–1000.

Index

Note: Page numbers of article titles are in **boldface** type.

Cardiol Clin 29 (2011) 315–318
doi:10.1016/S0733-8651(11)00028-2
0733-8651/11/$ – see front matter © 2011 Elsevier Inc. All rights reserved.

cardiology.theclinics.com

Printed and bound by CPI Group (UK) Ltd, Croydon, CR0 4YY

03/10/2024

01040355-0019